THE FAT TOOTH
RESTAURANT
& FAST-FOOD
FAT-GRAM COUNTER

Other Books by Joseph C. Piscatella

Don't Eat Your Heart Out Cookbook

Choices for a Healthy Heart

Controlling Your Fat Tooth

THE FAT TOOTH
RESTAURANT
& FAST-FOOD
FAT-GRAM COUNTER

By Joseph C. Piscatella
& Bernie Piscatella

WORKMAN PUBLISHING, NEW YORK

Library of Congress Cataloging-in-Publication Data

Piscatella, Joseph C.
The fat tooth fat gram counter / by Joseph C. Piscatella and Bernie Piscatella.
p.   cm.
ISBN 1-56305-149-4 (pbk.)
1. Food—Fat content—Tables.   2. Food—Caloric content—Tables.
I. Piscatella, Bernie.   II. Title.
TX551.P526   1993
641.1'4—dc20   91-50964
                          CIP

Workman books are available at special discount when purchased in bulk for special sales promotions as well as fund-raising or educational use. Special book excerpts or editions can also be created to specification. For details, contact the Special Sales Director at the address below.

Workman Publishing Company, Inc.
708 Broadway
New York, NY 10003

First printing March 1993
Manufactured in the United States of America

10 9 8 7 6 5 4

ACKNOWLEDGMENTS

There are many people to thank for their support and contribution in making this book a reality. In particular, we are grateful to Dr. Adam Drewnowski, Director of the Human Nutrition Center at the University of Michigan, for his research on "fat tooth" food cravings, and to Dr. Evette Hackman, a registered dietitian, for her critical analysis and valuable suggestions. Thanks also to Julie Hedrick for her tireless hours of nutritional analysis.

In addition, we'd like to thank Sally Barline, Kaye Bickford, Bette Kirk and Patty Brustkern for their valued suggestions. And finally, our thanks to Peter Workman and his faith in our work, and to Sally Kovalchick and Lynn Strong for their editorial expertise.

CONTENTS

VOLUME TWO: RESTAURANT GUIDE

The information in this book should not be construed as medical advice or instruction. Always consult your physician or other appropriate health professionals before making any dietary changes.

INTRODUCTION

If you want to stay within your fat budget and still live in the real world, you have to take restaurant food into consideration:

■ On average, Americans are eating out about three and a half times a week, often spending about 40% of their food budgets on restaurant fare.

■ There are now more than 82,000 fast-food restaurants in the United States.

■ The market for take-out food has surpassed $60 billion a year.

The Restaurant Food Lists are divided into two sections. The first deals with sit-down and take-out restaurant items. These items generally differ greatly from processed and homemade versions in terms of ingredients, preparation and cooking methods, and portion size. According to the USDA, the average serving of London broil (flank steak) at home, for example, is 3.5–4 ounces, or about 15 grams of fat. But in a restaurant the average serving is about 8 ounces, or 34 grams of fat! And that doesn't count any fat added in a sauce. Food items even change from restaurant to restaurant. Sometimes portion size is dictated simply by the size of the plates used—a restaurant with large plates tends to serve larger portions. Moreover, one restaurant might "dry-grill" an item, while another fries it in butter.

Recognizing the need for a restaurant guide and the wide variance in the fat content of restaurant items, we used information from the American Restaurant Association, *Restaurants and Institutions* magazine, individual restaurants and the American Culinary Institute. This information allowed us to create a list of the most popular and frequently ordered restaurant foods and the average fat contained in a normal serving of each item. Obviously, the list is neither endless nor exact. A chicken breast fillet served at your favorite local restaurant may not match up exactly to our average, but it will be close enough to give you a good idea of how that food item impacts your budget.

The second section deals with fast-food items, including burgers, chicken, fish, pizza, French fries and shakes, with nutritional information supplied by the individual food chains. Because most fast foods are precisely measured, there is a great degree of consistency to these items. Order a Big Mac at a McDonald's restaurant in Seattle or Atlanta and you'll get the same thing—in this instance, 26 grams of fat. Two slices of Domino's Pepperoni Pizza (16-inch, thin crust) yields 17 grams of fat, whether you buy and eat it in Detroit or in Los Angeles. So, from a monitoring standpoint, fast foods are very much like processed foods and make fat-budgeting easy.

It should also be noted that the figures for calories and fat have been rounded up or down for ease of calculation. If a food contains 88 to 92 calories, it is expressed in the lists as "90 calories"; if it contains 93 to 97 calories, it is shown as "95 calories." Fat grams are rounded off to the nearest whole number. If a food contains less than .5 grams of fat per serving, it is expressed as "0 grams."

As with processed foods, most people have favorite restaurant items they order over and over again. So, in the back of the book you'll find a section in which you can list your favorite and most frequently eaten restaurant foods. This customized list will save you time.

RESTAURANT STRATEGIES

Whether you're leisurely feasting at a four-star restaurant or simply rushing through your favorite fast-food outlet, there are strategies that are important to dietary control.

1. Know your personal fat budget and plan to stay on it. The budget is a guide-line for the day. Make a point of knowing how many grams of fat you have to "spend" before you go to the restaurant. Don't think of restaurant eating as being distinct from your at-home efforts to stay within your budget. Instead, see it as an extension of those efforts. Develop a healthy mindset. Don't think of eating out as a "special occasion" to eat whatever you want until you're stuffed. Understand how it fits in with your overall dietary plan. And if you do break your budget, redouble your efforts the following day—take a longer walk when you exercise, for example, and make sure all three meals are really low in fat. You can't undo the high-fat restaurant meal, but you can bring your dietary life back into balance so that your budget evens out over two days.

2. Choose a restaurant that prepares food you can eat. When someone asks "Where do you want to eat?" have in mind a list of restaurants where you know you can get low-fat items. Know which restaurants work for you. If you don't, your options may be severely limited. It's more difficult to make low-fat choices, for example, at a prime rib restaurant specializing in oversize portions or at a fried chicken/fish-and-chips fast-food restaurant. Think about what you want to order before you get to the restaurant. This will keep you from being caught offguard and ending up with a high-fat meal.

3. Don't set yourself up to overeat. If you skip meals all day long to "save calories" for a restaurant dinner, chances are good that you'll overeat. You'll arrive at the restaurant famished, so your resistance to fatty foods will be low. It's also easy to rationalize extras when you're starving. It's better to eat a low-fat breakfast and lunch to compensate for increased fat at dinner, but be sure to eat. A good tip is to be a little full before you order. You might want to have a glass of mineral water or fruit juice, a piece of fruit, or some raw vegetables and salsa an hour or so before dinner to take the edge off your hunger. Watch out for alcohol—it doesn't contain fat, but it may enhance your hunger. Have a Virgin Mary or other nonalcoholic cocktail before dinner. Not only will it help to hold your hunger in check, but it will keep you from feeling "deprived" of cocktail activities.

4. Make your desires known. Ask questions about how a food is prepared. Is it grilled? Fried? Steamed? Are fats added—oil, butter, cream or sour cream? The way to keep salmon from being served in a butter sauce, or vegetables served under melted cheese, is to tell the server what you want—and what you *don't* want. You, the customer, should have the final say in what you eat.

5. Look for key words on the menu. *Avoid the following:* buttery, butter sauce, sautéed, fried, pan-fried, crispy, creamed, cream sauce, in its own gravy, au gratin, in cheese sauce, escalloped, au lait, à la mode, au fromage, marinated, basted, prime, Hollandaise. *Choose instead:*

steamed, in broth, in its own juice, poached, garden fresh, roasted, broiled, stir-fried, lean.

6. Have some idea of serving size. The "normal" serving size in a restaurant is generally much greater than what you would get at home, so develop a mental picture of what a serving should be. For example, a 3-ounce portion of meat or fish is about the same size as the palm of a woman's hand, and 3 ounces of chicken is about one-half of a chicken breast. Three ounces of cooked rice equals one-half cup. Sometimes commercial packaging can help you to visualize serving size. A snack-size bag of potato or taco chips, for example, is just 1 ounce.

With this in mind, it isn't hard to see that the serving size in many restaurants may be twice that amount. Sandwiches made with mayonnaise at home usually contain 1 teaspoon per slice of bread, according to the USDA. But restaurants often slather mayonnaise on their sandwiches. If it's more than a thin spread, the sandwich may contain 1 to 1½ tablespoons. And remember, 1 tablespoon of mayonnaise contains 11 grams of fat! Salad dressing ladles at salad bars generally hold from 2 to 6 tablespoons of salad dressing. At the high end, that's enough dressing to equal the fat and calories of a Big Mac. And finally, most pasta dishes are calculated on a 9-ounce portion size—a 5-ounce portion of cooked pasta (visualize about 1 cup) and a 4-ounce portion of sauce (visualize about ½ cup). When is the last time a dish of pasta this size was served to you in a restaurant? Most restaurants actually serve 1½ to 2 times that amount. When eaten in too great a quantity, even low-fat foods can add up to excessive fat.

7. Use the food lists to preplan. The food lists allow you to preplan your meal before you arrive at the restaurant. There will be less temptation to deviate, you'll get what you want, and you'll stay within your budget.

ABBREVIATIONS

dia	= diameter	sm	= small
lb	= pound	tbsp	= tablespoon
lg	= large	tsp	= teaspoon
oz	= ounce	w/	= with
pkg	= package	w/o	= without
pkt	= packet	"	= inch

SIT-DOWN RESTAURANTS

Sit-down restaurants offer a variety of foods and preparation methods that can work to your benefit in restricting fat. Most restaurants want to please their customers and will make adjustments to their menu.

General Tips

Make basic low-fat choices. Seafood, for example, is usually lower in fat than red meat; a tomato-based sauce is lower than a cream-based sauce. Fried foods have more fat than broiled foods. Learn to distinguish high- from low-fat items on the menu.

■ When ordering your meal, consider preparation methods. Have your chicken, fish or meat grilled, broiled or steamed. Fried fish, for example, packs 18 to 20 grams of fat per 5-ounce fillet, while grilled fish has only 3 grams of fat.

■ Ask for substitutions to lower fat levels. Requesting a plain baked potato instead of

French fries, for example, will save 15 grams of fat. Other good substitutions are steamed vegetables for butter-topped and plain rice for rice pilaf.

■ Watch for fatty add-ons. Skip creamy sauces and dressings, or have them served on the side. Most cream-based sauces contain 9 to 13 grams of fat per 2 tablespoons. Keep fat levels down by controlling the amount of sauce or dressing you use.

■ Practice portion control. Remember, even if your order is low in fat, restaurant portions are generally twice what you should be eating. If you order beef, ask for the "petite," "queen" or "8-ounce" portion rather than the "king" or "16-ounce" cut. Consider sharing—one person can order an entrée while the other takes the salad bar. If you order a rich dessert, split it. One piece of chocolate cake shared among four people will give everyone a taste without destroying anyone's fat budget. And finally, don't feel compelled to eat everything just because you paid for it. Enjoy what you eat, but resist the urge to join the "Clean Plate Club."

■ Stay away from appetizers that are fried, drenched in oil or served with creamy dips. Nachos with guacamole, deep-fried mozzarella sticks, egg rolls and buffalo wings are good examples. Opt for fresh vegetables and salsa, seafood cocktail, oysters on the half shell, marinated vegetables, seviche, or low-fat soups.

■ Many restaurants automatically prepare vegetables with butter, margarine, oil or other fat. Ask for them without added fat. It makes no sense to have a low-fat entrée surrounded by fat-laden vegetables.

Meat, Poultry & Seafood

■ Ask for meat to be lean, well-trimmed and cooked in a low-fat manner. Order a small piece of sirloin, round steak or London broil, and ask that no butter or oil be used in preparation. Remember, the longer meat is cooked, the more time for fat to drip off. Order meat done to "medium" or "well-done" to reduce fat.

■ Avoid chicken that is fried, batter-dipped and fried, or served smothered with gravy. Order it baked, broiled or barbecued without the skin and with sauces served on the side. If your chicken is served with the skin on, remove the skin before eating.

■ Avoid fish and chips, and any seafood that is fried, deep-fried, breaded and fried, batter-dipped and fried, in a creamy sauce, served with cheese sauce, en casserole, Newburg, Thermidor, baked stuffed, and stuffed and rolled. Better choices are seafood that is broiled, blackened (Cajun style), in marinara sauce, in light wine sauce, grilled or mesquite-grilled, marinated, barbecued, stir-fried or steamed.

■ Skip fatty condiments such as butter, drawn butter, mayonnaise, tartar sauce and dill sauce. Better choices are low-sodium soy sauce, lemon juice, wine or vermouth, flavored vinegars and tomato salsa.

Salads

■ At the salad bar, skip tempting, high-fat extras such as bacon bits, cold cuts, egg yolks, olives and creamy pasta or potato salads. A typical 2-cup salad with all the high-fat extras can have as much as 30 grams of fat—as much as a cheeseburger.

■ A simple green salad is virtually fat-free and runs about 10 calories per ounce. But pour on a couple of tablespoons of dressing and fat/calories soar. Ask for diet and fat-free versions of salad dressings. Order dressing "on the side" and dip your fork in the dressing—you'll get all the flavor but very little of the fat. Don't overlook salsa as an alternative nonfat dressing.

■ Chef's salad, made with cheese, eggs, ham, roast beef and turkey roll bound together in a creamy dressing, is one of the fattest salads—about 800 calories and 65 grams of fat. Ask your server to skip the ham, beef and turkey roll in favor of skinless roast turkey, and substitute a low-fat variety of cheese (used sparingly) and low-fat dressing. You can save 50 grams of fat and 500 calories.

Ethnic Foods

■ In Italian restaurants, order veal piccata, chicken cacciatore, scampi sautéed in wine, or pizza with vegetable topping. Avoid sausage, cream sauces, salami, cheese, and bread drenched in oil (bruschetta) or butter (garlic bread).

Pasta can be a very healthful food or a nutritional disaster, depending on the sauce. Look for tomato-based sauces such as marinara, light red, vegetable and red seafood sauce. Avoid pasta in butter, cheese, oil, cream or bacon fat (pancetta) such as Alfredo or carbonara sauces, as well as those made with sausage. Pesto sauce is also rich in fat. Stuffed pastas—tortellini, ravioli, cannelloni, manicotti, lasagna—usually have high-fat filling.

■ The basic components of Mexican foods (lettuce, tomatoes, salsa, tortillas, pinto beans) start out low in fat, but preparation techniques as well as fatty "extras" can ruin the picture. Some pitfalls to watch for are cheese, sour cream and guacamole (all high in fat); refried beans (usually made with lard); deep-fried or crispy taco or salad shells, tortilla chips, nachos, chimichangas, flautas and quesadillas (all fried items). Better choices are soft-shell tacos or corn tortillas, burritos, enchiladas, fajitas, grilled chicken or fish, taco salads without the shell, and rice.

Lower-fat fillings can make a difference. The average beef-and-cheese enchilada, for instance, has 7 grams of fat; filled with chicken, the fat drops to 4 grams.

■ Chinese food offers a variety of low-fat options. Choose stir-fried or steamed dishes with vegetables, chicken and seafood. Duck, beef and pork are usually higher in fat. (Duck dishes are among the highest, so avoid Peking duck and crispy duck.) Skip items that are fried. Chinese appetizers (egg rolls, fried shrimp, fried chicken, fried wontons, fried raviolis) are among the worst. Better choices include steamed raviolis and roast pork strips.

Watch out for breaded and deep-fried foods such as sweet-and-sour dishes.

Choose white rice over fried rice, which contains added fat. Vegetable fried rice is preferable to pork or beef fried rice. Lo mein noodles are a better choice than fried noodles. Order the vegetable or shrimp varieties over those using pork or beef.

■ Thai food is generally light in calories and fat. Rice, noodles and vegetables dominate the menu, so it's easy to keep servings of meat and seafood moderate. Most entrées are stir-fried, steamed, boiled or barbecued. In addition to vegetables, entrées include shrimp, scallops, squid, clams, chicken, beef, pork and duck. (Avoid duck —it's too fatty.) Be certain that the restaurant stir-fries in vegetable oil, not lard. Watch out for appetizers such as fried or stuffed chicken wings, Thai rolls, tod mum and golden bags, which are fried or deep-fried.

It is not uncommon for peanuts, cashews or peanut sauces to be used in Thai cooking. Avoid such dishes because of high fat content.

Many Thai dishes call for coconut milk, which has about 48 grams of fat per cup. Stay clear of coconut-milk dishes, such as curry or chicken coconut soup. If you do order curry, a Thai specialty, consider sharing it with your dinner partner.

■ Japanese steak houses offer an Americanized version of Japanese food—one that is not low in fat. Authentic Japanese cooking, however, is centered on low-fat rice and vegetables and uses little or no fat in cooking. Most of the fat in Japanese dishes comes from the food itself, so order fish, shellfish and poultry over beef or pork. Low-fat preparation methods include steaming, boiling and simmering. Methods to avoid are tempura, agemono and katsu. Good choices are sukiyaki, sushi, sashimi, Japanese vegetables, chicken and fish teriyaki, and rice and noodles.

■ Look for French/Continental restaurants that specialize in the foods of southern France (Provençal), which use seafood, vegetables, wine and olive oil rather than the meat, sausage, goose, lard, goose fat, butter, cream and fatty sauces featured in northern French cooking. Avoid quiche, goose or duck pâté, organ meats, rich sauces such as Béarnaise and Hollandaise, croissants and pastry. Smarter choices are poached or broiled fish, salade Niçoise, coq au vin, bouillabaisse and nouvelle cuisine preparations of lean meat and poultry.

APPETIZERS

	AMOUNT	CALORIES	FAT-GRAMS	% FAT
Antipasto platter (lettuce, salami, prosciutto, cheese, anchovies, egg, tomato, onion, olives, celery	1 serving	230	15	59
Artichoke, fresh	1 med	55	0	0
Asparagus w/ prosciutto	3 spears	55	2	33
BBQ pork w/ seeds & hot mustard	2 oz	215	14	59
BBQ ribs	3 oz	390	27	63
Beef Chiang Mai	1 serving	125	8	58
Belgian pâté	2 oz	150	14	83
Bruschetta (broiled French or Italian bread, olive oil)	1 slice	240	20	75
Calamari, fried	5 oz	215	11	48
Caponata	6 oz	185	14	68
Caviar	1 tbsp	40	2	43
w/ hard-cooked eggs, chopped onions & chives		140	5	32

17

	AMOUNT	CALORIES	FAT-GRAMS	% FAT
Celery stuffed w/ blue cheese	2 stalks	105	9	76
Celery stuffed w/ olives & cream cheese	2 stalks	85	7	74
Cheese:				
Baked chèvre w/ French roll	1 serving	275	11	36
Buffalo mozzarella w/ tomatoes, basil, black olives & olive oil	3 oz	345	37	96
Cheese & crab tarts	2	400	28	63
Cheese bagel bites	1	30	2	60
Cheese board (2 oz cheese, 2 oz crackers	1 serving	510	34	59
Cheese nuggets (½-oz balls)	2	165	9	49
Cheese sticks	1 oz	160	11	62
Cherry tomato stuffed w/ cream cheese	1	35	3	75
Fried cheese (2½ x ½ x ½)	1 stick	75	5	59
Fried cheese kabob	1	65	4	55
Fried mozzarella w/ marinara sauce	3 oz	340	22	58
Marinated mozzarella	1 oz	150	14	85
Pesto cheese torta (pesto, mascarpone, ricotta)	2.5 oz	155	13	75
Ricotta cheese spread	1 tbsp	45	2	40
Swiss cheese tartlets	2	435	33	68

	AMOUNT	CALORIES	FAT-GRAMS	% FAT
Chicken:				
BBQ chicken wing (2 oz)	1	130	6	41
Cajun chicken wings	1 wing	130	7	49
Chicken liver pâté	¼ cup	295	26	79
Chicken liver pâte on 1 slice toast	1 serving	162	8	36
Chicken livers wrapped in bacon (rumaki)	2	105	5	44
Chicken nuggets (3.5 oz each)	4	240	14	52
Chicken wings, batter-dipped, fried	1.7 oz	160	11	62
Chicken wings teriyaki	2 oz	155	6	35
Chopped chicken liver & eggs	¼ cup	210	17	72
Ginger chicken wings	1 wing	170	13	69
Chili con queso	¼ cup	200	16	73
w/ 1 oz chips		340	22	58
Chinese crab claws	2	150	8	49
Chips:				
Chips & salsa (1 cup chips, ¼ cup salsa)	1 serving	215	11	51
Nacho chips	1 oz	150	8	48
Nachos, cheese (1 oz chips, 2 oz sauce)	1 serving	310	13	38

	AMOUNT	CALORIES	FAT-GRAMS	% FAT
Nachos, deluxe (1 oz chips, 2 oz sauce, ground beef, refried beans, cheese)	1 serving	430	19	40
Nachos Grande (ground beef, tomatoes, olives, lettuce, cheese, sour cream, 2 oz chips)	1 serving	635	39	55
Potato chips	1 oz	150	10	60
Taco chips	1 oz	140	7	47
Tortilla chips	1 oz	140	6	38
w/ ¼ cup salsa		160	7	39
Clams:				
Clams on half shell	6	150	1	6
Deviled clams	1 ramekin	360	14	35
Fried clams	6 oz	380	20	47
Steamed clams (in shells)	1 lb	265	8	28
w/ olive oil & lemon		335	21	56
Cocktail meatballs	3	150	9	54
Codfish balls	1 ball	50	3	55
Crab:				
Chinese crab claws	2	150	8	49
Crab & cheese tarts	2	400	28	63
Crab claws	6 oz	145	1	6
Crab Imperial	1 ramekin	140	7	44
Crabmeat cocktail	1 serving	130	2	14
Crab pillows	3	120	6	46

	Amount	Calories	Fat-Grams	% Fat
Dips:				
Avocado	¼ cup	100	8	72
Bacon & horseradish	¼ cup	100	10	90
Blue cheese	¼ cup	125	9	65
Clam dip	¼ cup	140	10	63
Creamy cucumber	¼ cup	100	8	72
French onion	¼ cup	120	8	60
Garlic	¼ cup	120	8	60
Gaucamole	¼ cup	80	8	88
Jalapeño	¼ cup	120	10	75
Nacho cheese	¼ cup	100	4	36
Picante sauce	¼ cup	40	0	0
Egg rolls:				
Crab-filled	1	155	10	58
Ham-filled	1	135	8	54
Meatless	1	100	6	52
Pork-filled	1	170	8	42
Pork & shrimp-filled	1	160	9	51
Shrimp-filled	1	190	6	29
Vegetable-filled	1	120	6	45
Eggs:				
Deviled	1 egg	140	12	77
Pickled	1 egg	85	6	64
Empanadas	2	195	14	64
Escargots w/ butter sauce	3 oz	450	25	50
Finger sandwiches:				
Cheese	1 sq	45	2	40
Cucumber	1 sq	30	1	30
Cucumber & shrimp	1 sq	45	2	40
Ham	1 sq	45	2	40
Watercress	1 sq	30	1	30

	AMOUNT	CALORIES	FAT-GRAMS	% FAT
Fruit:				
Citrus cocktail	½ cup	55	0	0
w/ avocado		70	2	26
Fruit cocktail	½ cup	65	0	0
Fruit platter				
w/ 2 oz cheese	1 serving	310	18	52
Mandarin orange/				
banana cocktail	½ cup	45	0	0
Melon & prosciutto	1 wedge	35	1	26
Melon cocktail	½ cup	30	0	0
in syrup		85	0	0
Peach & green grape				
cocktail	½ cup	40	0	0
Gyoza	4	255	9	32
Ham phyllo roll	1	75	3	36
Kielbasa in fondue				
(6 oz)	1 serving	410	33	72
Lobster cocktail	1 serving	130	2	14
Mushrooms:				
Bread-stuffed	1	35	2	51
Cheese-stuffed	1	45	3	63
Marinated	2	15	1	60
Wrapped in bacon	2	50	4	69
Mushroom spread				
w/ 2 crackers	1 serving	85	2	21
Mussels, steamed				
(in olive oil,				
garlic, tomatoes)	1 doz	330	12	33
Nachos. *See* Chips.				
Nuts:				
Almonds				
Dry roasted	1 oz	170	15	80
Honey roasted	1 oz	170	13	69
Cashews	1 oz	170	13	69

	AMOUNT	CALORIES	FAT-GRAMS	% FAT
Mixed nuts	1 oz	170	13	69
Peanuts				
Dry roasted	1 oz	160	14	79
Honey roasted	1 oz	160	13	73
Oil roasted	1 oz	170	15	79
Olives:				
Green				
Medium	10	45	5	100
Large	10	65	7	100
Giant	10	76	8	100
Ripe (extra-large)	10	61	6	100
Stuffed, rolled				
w/ bacon	2	50	4	75
Onion rings	2	80	5	55
Oysters:				
Angels on horseback				
(oysters wrapped				
in bacon)	1	60	4	61
Oysters on half-shell	6	120	2	15
Oysters Rockefeller	6	355	26	66
Oyster shooter	1 med	40	1	22
Pâtés:				
Belgian pâté	2 oz	150	14	83
Chicken liver pâté	¼ cup	295	26	79
Pickled herring	1.75 oz	130	6	14
Piroshki, ham & egg	2	320	23	64
Piroshki, Russian	2	340	24	64
Pizza bites	2 pcs	65	4	55
Pizza bread (1 slice				
bread, 1 oz cheese)	1 serving	200	10	45
Popcorn:				
Air-popped	1 cup	30	0	0
Coated w/ sugar				
syrup	1 cup	135	1	7

	AMOUNT	CALORIES	FAT-GRAMS	% FAT
Oil-popped	1 cup	55	3	49
w/ ½ tsp butter		70	5	62
Potatoes:				
French fries	1 potato	240	12	45
Fried potato skins	1 med potato	220	12	50
Potato chips	1 oz	150	9	60
Spiral fries	1 med potato	285	14	44
Pot stickers	4	255	9	32
Pretzels	1 oz	110	1	8
Rumaki	2	105	5	44
Smoked salmon	3 oz	100	4	36
w/ 2 oz cream cheese, capers, onions		315	24	68
Sauerkraut balls	2	120	5	37
Seafood nuggets	2 oz	130	8	55
Shrimp:				
BBQ jumbo shrimp	4 lg	70	1	13
Jumbo prawn cocktail	6 prawns	155	2	12
Peel & eat shrimp	3 oz	90	1	10
Shrimp cocktail	4 shrimp	105	1	9
Shrimp wrapped w/ bacon	1 shrimp	30	2	60
Spring rolls	1	130	8	55
Squash blossoms stuffed w/ prosciutto, mozzarella & ricotta	4	170	12	64
Steak tartar	4 oz	545	39	64
Sushi w/ vegetables	4.5 oz	180	1	5

	AMOUNT	CALORIES	FAT GRAMS	% FAT
Szechuan pork & seeds w/ hot mustard	2 oz	215	14	59
Tuna:				
Broiled tuna Hawaiian on 1 slice bread	1 serving	105	6	52
Deviled tuna cheeseburger (petite bun)	1	235	11	42
Turkey aiguillettes	2 oz	210	13	56
Vegetable antipasto platter	1 serving	225	20	80
Vegetables:				
Batter-fried	¾ cup	150	7	42
Raw (w/ olive oil)	1 serving	225	20	80
Wontons, filled	4	255	9	32
Wonton skins, fried	½ cup	110	8	65
Zucchini Carpaccio	1 serving	280	27	87

BEVERAGES

ALCOHOLIC BEVERAGES

	AMOUNT	CALORIES	FAT-GRAMS	% FAT
BEER, ALE & MALT LIQUOR				
Ale	12 fl oz	155	0	0
Beer	12 fl oz	145	0	0
Light	12 fl oz	100	0	0
Malt liquor	12 fl oz	150	0	0
Amstel Light	12 fl oz	95	0	0
Anheuser-Busch	12 fl oz	155	0	0
Natural Light	12 fl oz	110	0	0
Beck's	12 fl oz	145	0	0
Dark	12 fl oz	155	0	0
Black Horse	12 fl oz	160	0	0
Black Label	12 fl oz	135	0	0
Blatz Ale	12 fl oz	155	0	0
Blatz Beer	12 fl oz	140	0	0
Budweiser	12 fl oz	145	0	0
Bud Light	12 fl oz	110	0	0
Busch	12 fl oz	145	0	0
Light	12 fl oz	110	0	0
Champale Malt Liquor	12 fl oz	170	0	0
Colt 45 Malt Liquor	12 fl oz	155	0	0

	AMOUNT	CALORIES	FAT-GRAMS	% FAT
Coors	12 fl oz	140	0	0
Light	12 fl oz	105	0	0
Corona Light	12 fl oz	105	0	0
Hamm's Light	12 fl oz	95	0	0
Heidelberg Light	12 fl oz	115	0	0
Heileman				
Old Style	12 fl oz	145	0	0
Light	12 fl oz	100	0	0
Special Export	12 fl oz	155	0	0
Light	12 fl oz	115	0	0
Heineken	12 fl oz	150	0	0
Knickerbocker	12 fl oz	140	0	0
Lite Genuine Draft	12 fl oz	100	0	0
Michelob	12 fl oz	160	0	0
Classic Dark	12 fl oz	165	0	0
Light	12 fl oz	135	0	0
Mickey's Malt Liquor	12 fl oz	155	0	0
Miller				
High Life	12 fl oz	150	0	0
Lite	12 fl oz	95	0	0
Milwaukee's Best,				
Light	12 fl oz	100	0	0
Molson Light	12 fl oz	110	0	0
Old Milwaukee,				
Light	12 fl oz	120	0	0
Old Style Light	12 fl oz	115	0	0
Olympia Gold Light	12 fl oz	70	0	0
Pabst Blue Ribbon	12 fl oz	145	0	0
Light	12 fl oz	70	0	0
Piels Light	12 fl oz	135	0	0
Rainier	12 fl oz	140	0	0
Rheingold	12 fl oz	150	0	0
Light	12 fl oz	95	0	0
Schaefer Light	12 fl oz	110	0	0

BEVERAGES

	AMOUNT	CALORIES	FAT-GRAMS	% FAT
Schlitz Light	12 fl oz	95	0	0
Schmidt's	12 fl oz	150	0	0
Light	12 fl oz	95	0	0
Stroh's	12 fl oz	145	0	0
Tiger Head Ale	12 fl oz	165	0	0

DISTILLED LIQUOR

(The higher the proof, the greater the amount of alcohol and calories.)

	AMOUNT	CALORIES	FAT-GRAMS	% FAT
Proof				
80	1 fl oz	67	0	0
84	1 fl oz	70	0	0
86	1 fl oz	72	0	0
90	1 fl oz	75	0	0
94	1 fl oz	78	0	0
97	1 fl oz	81	0	0
100	1 fl oz	83	0	0
Bloody Mary	5 fl oz	120	0	0
Bourbon & soda	5 fl oz	120	0	0
Brandy Alexander	5 fl oz	275	9	29
Brandy cream	4 fl oz	150	7	42
Campari & soda	5 fl oz	120	0	0
Daiquiri:	2.5 fl oz	90	0	0
Banana	4 fl oz	145	0	0
Peach	4 fl oz	110	0	0
Strawberry	4 fl oz	145	0	0
Gin:				
90-proof	1 jigger	110	0	0
94-proof	1 jigger	115	0	0
100-proof	1 jigger	125	0	0
Gin & tonic	7.5 fl oz	170	0	0
Glögg	4 fl oz	190	2	9
Golden Cadillac	4 fl oz	230	7	27
Grasshopper	4 fl oz	230	7	27

	AMOUNT	CALORIES	FAT-GRAMS	% FAT
Highball	7.5 fl oz	165	0	0
Hot buttered rum	6 fl oz	255	9	32
Irish coffee	6 fl oz	280	11	35
Manhattan	2 fl oz	130	0	0
Margarita	4 fl oz	250	0	0
Martini	2.5 fl oz	155	0	0
Mexican Sunset	5 fl oz	200	0	0
Mint julep	10 fl oz	210	0	0
Old-fashioned	2.5 fl oz	130	0	0
Piña colada	4.5 fl oz	260	3	10
Rum:				
80-proof	1 jigger	100	0	0
94-proof	1 jigger	115	0	0
100-proof	1 jigger	125	0	0
Scotch	1 jigger	115	0	0
Screwdriver	7 fl oz	175	0	0
Sloe gin fizz	2.5 fl oz	130	0	0
Tequila	1 jigger	115	0	0
Tequila Sunrise	5 fl oz	200	0	0
Tom Collins	5 fl oz	120	0	0
Velvet Hammer	4 fl oz	230	7	27
Vodka:				
94-proof	1 jigger	115	0	0
100-proof	1 jigger	125	0	0
Whiskey:				
94-proof	1 jigger	115	0	0
100-proof	1 jigger	125	0	0
Whiskey sour	4 fl oz	170	0	0

LIQUEURS

Amaretto	1.5 fl oz	120	0	0
Anisette	1.5 fl oz	150	0	0
Apricot brandy	1.5 fl oz	120	0	0
B&B	1.5 fl oz	140	0	0

	AMOUNT	CALORIES	FAT-GRAMS	% FAT
Benedictine	1.5 fl oz	140	0	0
Brandy	1.5 fl oz	105	0	0
Cherry Heering	1.5 fl oz	120	0	0
Coffee liqueur:				
53-proof	1.5 fl oz	175	0	0
63-proof	1.5 fl oz	160	0	0
Coffee w/ Cream	1.5 fl oz	155	7	40
Crème d'Amande	1.5 fl oz	150	0	0
Crème de Banane	1.5 fl oz	145	0	0
Crème de Cacao	1.5 fl oz	150	0	0
Crème de Cassis	1.5 fl oz	120	0	0
Crème de Menthe	1.5 fl oz	190	0	0
Curaçao	1.5 fl oz	110	0	0
Drambuie	1.5 fl oz	165	0	0
Grand Marnier	1.5 fl oz	120	0	0
Kirsch	1.5 fl oz	125	0	0
Peppermint				
schnapps	1.5 fl oz	125	0	0
Pernod	1.5 fl oz	120	0	0
Rock & rye	1.5 fl oz	140	0	0
Sloe gin	1.5 fl oz	125	0	0
Southern Comfort	1.5 fl oz	180	0	0
Tía Maria	1.5 fl oz	140	0	0
Triple Sec	1.5 fl oz	120	0	0

WINES

	AMOUNT	CALORIES	FAT-GRAMS	% FAT
Beaujolais	4 fl oz	95	0	0
Bordeaux, red	4 fl oz	95	0	0
Burgundy:				
Red	4 fl oz	95	0	0
Sparkling	4 fl oz	115	0	0
White	4 fl oz	90	0	0
Cabernet				
Sauvignon	4 fl oz	90	0	0

	AMOUNT	CALORIES	FAT-GRAMS	% FAT
Chablis	4 fl oz	85	0	0
Emerald, gold, pink	4 fl oz	100	0	0
Champagne:				
Brut, pink	4 fl oz	100	0	0
Extra-dry	4 fl oz	105	0	0
Chardonnay	4 fl oz	90	0	0
Chenin Blanc	4 fl oz	85	0	0
Chianti	4 fl oz	100	0	0
Cold Duck	4 fl oz	110	0	0
Dessert	4 fl oz	180	0	0
Dubonnet	4 fl oz	160	0	0
French Colombard	4 fl oz	90	0	0
Liebfraumilch	4 fl oz	85	0	0
Madeira	4 fl oz	160	0	0
Muscatel	3.5 fl oz	160	0	0
Port:				
Ruby	4 fl oz	185	0	0
Tawny	4 fl oz	185	0	0
White	4 fl oz	170	0	0
Rhine	4 fl oz	95	0	0
Rhone	4 fl oz	95	0	0
Riesling	4 fl oz	90	0	0
Rosé	4 fl oz	95	0	0
Sauterne	4 fl oz	115	0	0
Sauvignon Blanc	4 fl oz	80	0	0
Sherry				
Cream	4 fl oz	115	0	0
Dry	4 fl oz	110	0	0
Sweet wines	4 fl oz	165	0	0
Sylvaner	4 fl oz	90	0	0
Table wines				
Red	3.5 fl oz	75	0	0
Rosé	3.5 fl oz	75	0	0
White	3.5 fl oz	70	0	0

	AMOUNT	CALORIES	FAT-GRAMS	% FAT
Tokay	4 fl oz	165	0	0
Vermouth				
Dry	4 fl oz	135	0	0
Sweet	4 fl oz	170	0	0
Wine cooler	12 fl oz	190	0	0
Wine spritzer	5 fl oz	60	0	0
Zinfandel				
Red	4 fl oz	90	0	0
White	4 fl oz	80	0	0

NONALCOHOLIC BEVERAGES

CARBONATED BEVERAGES

	AMOUNT	CALORIES	FAT-GRAMS	% FAT
Drink mixers:				
Bitter lemon	6 fl oz	75	0	0
Club soda	6 fl oz	0	0	0
Collins mixer	6 fl oz	60	0	0
Ginger ale	6 fl oz	70	0	0
Diet	6 fl oz	5	0	0
Grapefruit	6 fl oz	80	0	0
Lemon-lime	6 fl oz	75	0	0
Diet	6 fl oz	0	0	0
Lemon sour	6 fl oz	75	0	0
Quinine water	6 fl oz	70	0	0
Seltzer, plain & flavored	6 fl oz	0	0	0
Sour mixer	6 fl oz	70	0	0
Tonic water	6 fl oz	65	0	0
Diet	6 fl oz	5	0	0
Vodka mixer	6 fl oz	70	0	0
Mineral & bottled water	6 fl oz	0	0	0

	AMOUNT	CALORIES	FAT-GRAMS	% FAT
Soft drinks & sodas:				
Apple	6 fl oz	90	0	0
Diet	6 fl oz	10	0	0
Black cherry	6 fl oz	90	0	0
Diet	6 fl oz	5	0	0
Cherry cola	6 fl oz	80	0	0
Diet	6 fl oz	0	0	0
Cherry	6 fl oz	85	0	0
Diet	6 fl oz	0	0	0
Cola	6 fl oz	80	0	0
Diet	6 fl oz	0	0	0
Cream soda	6 fl oz	95	0	0
Diet	6 fl oz	0	0	0
Grape	6 fl oz	90	0	0
Diet	6 fl oz	5	0	0
7-Up	6 fl oz	80	0	0
Diet	6 fl oz	0	0	0
Orange	6 fl oz	100	0	0
Diet	6 fl oz	5	0	0
Punch				
Fruit	4 fl oz	65	0	0
Ice cream	4 fl oz	125	4	29
Lime ice ginger ale	4 fl oz	65	0	0
Rhubarb	4 fl oz	120	0	0
Sangría	4 fl oz	115	0	0
Sherbet	4 fl oz	125	1	7
Slushy	4 fl oz	75	0	0
Spiked	4 fl oz	100	0	0
Root beer	6 fl oz	85	0	0
Diet	6 fl oz	0	0	0
Float	12 fl oz	185	7	34
Strawberry	6 fl oz	90	0	0
Diet	6 fl oz	0	0	0

	AMOUNT	CALORIES	FAT-GRAMS	% FAT
NONCARBONATED BEVERAGES				
Cocoa/chocolate, hot:				
Prepared w/ water	6 fl oz	50	0	0
Diet	6 fl oz	20	0	0
Prepared w/				
1% milk	6 fl oz	150	3	18
2% milk	6 fl oz	165	5	27
Skim milk	6 fl oz	135	2	10
Whole milk	6 fl oz	180	7	35
Coffee & coffee beverages:				
Black regular				
Brewed	6 fl oz	5	0	0
Instant, powder	6 fl oz	5	0	0
Additions				
Half-and-half	1 tbsp	20	2	90
Light table cream	1 tbsp	30	3	90
Milk				
Skim	1 tbsp	5	0	0
Whole	1 tbsp	10	.5	45
Nondairy lightener				
Liquid	1 tbsp	20	2	90
Powdered	1 tsp	10	1	90
Sugar	1 tsp	15	0	0
	1 lump	15	0	0
	1 pkt	25	0	0
Sugar substitutes	1 pkt	0–5	0	0
Café au lait	6 fl oz	60	3	30
Caffe con latte				
Small				
w/ skim milk	8 fl oz	70	.4	5
w/ whole milk	8 fl oz	130	8	52

	AMOUNT	CALORIES	FAT-GRAMS	% FAT
Medium				
w/ skim milk	14 fl oz	110	.6	5
w/ whole milk	14 fl oz	205	12	52
Large				
w/ skim milk	16 fl oz	140	.7	5
w/ whole milk	16 fl oz	260	15	52
Cappuccino				
Small				
w/ skim milk	8 fl oz	30	.2	6
w/ whole milk	8 fl oz	55	3	48
Medium				
w/ skim milk	14 fl oz	50	.3	6
w/ whole milk	14 fl oz	95	5	48
Large				
w/ skim milk	16 fl oz	60	.4	6
w/ whole milk	16 fl oz	130	7	48
Iced coffee	8 fl oz	40	2	45
Mocha				
Small				
w/ skim milk	8 fl oz	150	6	35
w/ whole milk	8 fl oz	195	11	53
Medium				
w/ skim milk	14 fl oz	205	8	35
w/ whole milk	14 fl oz	285	17	53
Large				
w/ skim milk	16 fl oz	260	10	35
w/ whole milk	16 fl oz	355	21	53
Eggnog	8 fl oz	410	28	62
Chocolate	8 fl oz	450	26	52
Fruit drinks:				
Black cherry cooler	8 fl oz	90	0	0
Cranberry juice cocktail	6 fl oz	110	0	0
Fruit juice float	8 fl oz	205	7	30

	AMOUNT	CALORIES	FAT-GRAMS	% FAT
Fruit punch	6 fl oz	85	0	0
Lemonade	8 fl oz	100	0	0
Limeade	8 fl oz	100	0	0
Fruit juices:				
Apple	6 fl oz	90	0	0
Apple cider	6 fl oz	90	0	0
Apple-cranberry	6 fl oz	85	0	0
Apple-raspberry	6 fl oz	100	0	0
Cherry	6 fl oz	100	0	0
Cranapple	6 fl oz	120	0	0
Cranberry	6 fl oz	100	0	0
Cranberry-grape	6 fl oz	130	0	0
Grape	6 fl oz	110	0	0
Grapefruit	6 fl oz	70	0	0
Lemon	2 tbsp	10	0	0
Lime	2 tbsp	10	0	0
Orange	6 fl oz	90	0	0
Orange-grapefruit	6 fl oz	80	0	0
Orange-pineapple	6 fl oz	80	0	0
Peach	6 fl oz	100	0	0
Pineapple	6 fl oz	100	0	0
Pineapple-grapefruit	6 fl oz	90	0	0
Prune	6 fl oz	120	0	0
Milk:				
1% milk	8 fl oz	105	3	26
2% milk	8 fl oz	120	5	38
Buttermilk	8 fl oz	100	2	18
Skim milk	8 fl oz	85	0	0
Whole milk	8 fl oz	150	8	48
Milk drinks:				
Chocolate milk				
Prepared w/				
1% milk	8 fl oz	160	3	17
2% milk	8 fl oz	180	5	25

	Amount	Calories	Fat-Grams	% Fat
Skim milk	8 fl oz	160	0	0
Whole milk	8 fl oz	210	8	34
Milk shake				
Chocolate	10 fl oz	360	11	28
Malt	10 fl oz	405	20	44
Strawberry	10 fl oz	320	8	23
Vanilla	10 fl oz	315	8	23
Strawberry-flavored				
milk	8 fl oz	210	8	34
Yogurt smoothie	8 fl oz	135	3	20
Tea:				
Iced pineapple tea	6 fl oz	80	0	0
Iced tea	6 fl oz	5	0	0
Regular tea				
Bag	6 fl oz	0	0	0
Brewed	6 fl oz	0	0	0
Instant	6 fl oz	0	0	0
Sugar-free	6 fl oz	0	0	0
Additions				
Half-and-half	1 tbsp	20	2	90
Honey	1 tsp	20	0	0
Lemon	1 pc	0	0	0
Milk				
Skim	1 tbsp	5	0	0
Whole milk	1 tbsp	10	.5	45
Nondairy				
lightener				
Liquid	1 tbsp	20	2	90
Powdered	1 tsp	10	1	90
Sugar	1 tsp	15	0	0
	1 lump	15	0	0
	1 pkt	25	0	0
Sugar				
substitutes	1 pkt	0–5	0	0

	AMOUNT	CALORIES	FAT-GRAMS	% FAT
Russian tea	6 fl oz	100	0	0
Spiced tea	6 fl oz	100	0	0
Texas red-eye tea	6 fl oz	45	0	0
Vegetable juices:				
Carrot juice	6 fl oz	75	0	0
Tomato juice	6 fl oz	30	0	0
Spicy	6 fl oz	40	0	0
Vegetable juice				
cocktail	6 fl oz	35	0	0
Spicy	6 fl oz	40	0	0

BREADS

	AMOUNT	CALORIES	FAT-GRAMS	% FAT
Apple kuchen	1	290	12	37
Bagels:				
Cinnamon & raisin	1 lg	240	2	7
Onion	1 lg	230	1	4
Plain	1 lg	230	1	4
Biscuits:				
Biscuit & sausage (2.6 oz sausage, ¼ cup gravy)	1 serving	535	38	64
Biscuit, meat & gravy	1 serving	480	31	58
Biscuit w/ ¼ cup gravy	1 serving	275	14	46
Cheese biscuit	1	230	11	43
Scone	1	363	14	33
Shortcake biscuit	1	300	16	48
Southern biscuit	1	195	8	37
Bread:				
Buttermilk bread	1 slice	75	2	24
Cheese bread	1 slice	180	10	50
Chorizo bread	1 slice	345	21	55
Country oat bread	1 slice	90	2	20
Cracked wheat bread	1 slice	70	2	26

	AMOUNT	CALORIES	FAT-GRAMS	% FAT
Dark wheat bread	1 slice	80	1	11
Dill rye bread	1 slice	80	1	11
English mead bread	1 slice	115	2	15
Falafel (1 oz)	1 patty	57	3	47
Focaccia	1 slice	175	6	31
w/ vegetable topping & cheese		295	12	37
French bread	1 slice	70	1	13
Green chili bread	1 slice	160	2	11
Grilled herb flatbread		265	13	44
Honey wheat bread	1 slice	70	1	13
Irish soda bread	1 slice	145	2	12
Italian bread	1 slice	70	1	13
w/ tomato, basil & mozzarella		180	5	25
Italian bomba bread	1 wedge	360	12	30
Italian rosemary bread	1 slice	75	1	12
Multi-grain bread	1 slice	80	1	11
Pita bread (2 oz)	1 pocket	160	1	6
Pumpernickel	1 slice	80	1	11
Raisin bread	1 slice	70	1	13
Rye bread	1 slice	60	1	14
Sourdough bread	1 slice	70	1	13
Tenderfoot bread	1 slice	270	12	40
White bread	1 slice	80	1	11
Whole wheat 100% stone ground	1 slice	70	1	13
Bread spreads:				
Apple butter	1 tbsp	35	0	0
Apple jelly	1 tbsp	50	0	0

	AMOUNT	CALORIES	FAT-GRAMS	% FAT
Butter (1 pat)	1 tsp	36	4	100
Grape jelly	1 tbsp	50	0	0
Honey	1 tbsp	65	0	0
Jam, all flavors	1 tbsp	50	0	0
Jam, sugar-free	1 tbsp	15	0	0
Jelly, all flavors	1 tbsp	50	0	0
Margarine (1 pat)	1 tsp	34	4	100
Whipped	1 tsp	70	7	100
Orange marmalade	1 tbsp	50	0	0
Peach butter	1 tbsp	35	0	0
Preserves, all flavors	1 tbsp	50	0	0
Bread sticks:				
Italian bread sticks	1 stick	45	1	19
Onion bread sticks	1 stick	40	1	23
Plain bread sticks	1 stick	40	1	23
Sesame bread sticks	1 stick	50	2	36
Soft bread sticks	1 stick	70	2	26
Soft cheddar sticks	1 each	100	6	53
Soft pretzels (1 oz each)		125	2	14
Brioche	1 slice	135	5	33
Bruschetta w/ olives & tomatoes	1 slice	240	20	75
Buns:				
Chinese steamed bun	1	190	8	38
Hamburger bun	1	120	2	15
Hot dog bun	1	120	2	15
Kaiser bun	1	185	3	15
Cheese bread (1 slice bread, 1 oz cheese)	1 serving	180	10	50
Corn bread (4" x 4")	1 serving	280	11	36
Corn fritter	1	60	2	29

	AMOUNT	CALORIES	FAT-GRAMS	% FAT
Crackers:				
Chicken in a Basket	7 crackers	70	4	51
Cracked wheat crackers	4	110	4	33
Hearty wheat crackers	4	100	4	36
Lahvosh	1	30	1	30
Melba toast cracker	1	20	0	0
Oyster crackers	16	60	2	30
Ritz crackers	4	70	4	51
Rye crisps	4	90	0	0
Saltines	2	25	1	36
Triscuits	7	145	5	31
Toasted sesame cracker	1	30	0	0
Wheatsworth crackers	5	70	3	38
Wheat Thins	7	80	4	45
Crepes (unfilled)	2	150	7	42
Croissant	1	235	12	46
Croutons	½ oz	70	3	30
Doughnuts:				
Cake-type doughnut				
Plain (1.5 oz)	1	165	8	44
Sugared (1.6 oz)	1	185	8	39
Chocolate-covered doughnut	1	180	10	50
Jelly-filled doughnut (2.3 oz)	1	225	9	36
Raised doughnut, plain	1	120	4	30
Sopapilla	1	170	7	37
English muffin	1	130	1	7
French toast	2 slices	255	7	24

	AMOUNT	CALORIES	FAT-GRAMS	% FAT
Fruit square	1	250	3	11
Garlic bread	1 slice	110	7	56
Green chili bread	1 slice	160	2	11
Gruyère puff ring	⅛ ring	205	13	57
Hush puppies (1.5 oz each)	2	140	5	32
Melba toast (chef-prepared)				
Anchovy	1 slice	110	5	40
Cheese	1 slice	105	5	43
Garlic	1 slice	165	6	32
Herb	1 slice	165	6	32
Peanut butter	1 slice	110	5	40
Plain	1 slice	115	6	46
Sesame	1 slice	115	6	46
Muffins:				
Regular size (1.5 oz)				
Apple	1	205	7	30
Blueberry	1	195	10	46
Bran	1	125	6	33
Bran raisin	1	190	6	28
Corn	1	180	7	35
Extra-large size (5 oz)				
Bran	1	405	21	44
Poppy	1	495	22	39
Pancakes (6"):				
Banana pancakes	2	320	11	31
Blueberry pancakes	2	310	11	32
Buckwheat pancakes	2	275	6	20
Buttermilk pancakes	2	330	10	27
Cherry pancakes	2	335	11	29
Cornmeal pancakes	3	145	1	6
Johnnycakes	2	175	3	15
Plain pancakes	2	340	10	26

BREADS

	AMOUNT	CALORIES	FAT-GRAMS	% FAT
Pancake & waffle toppings:				
Butter	1 tbsp	100	11	100
	1 tsp/pat	35	4	100
Whipped	1 tbsp	60	7	100
Margarine				
Soft	1 tbsp	100	11	100
Stick	1 tbsp	100	11	100
	1 tsp/pat	35	4	100
Syrups				
Genovese	1 tbsp	50	0	0
Log Cabin				
Syrup	1 oz	99	0	0
Buttered	1 oz	106	0	0
Country				
Kitchen	1 oz	101	0	0
Lite	1 oz	61	0	0
Maple Honey	1 oz	106	0	0
Raspberry	1 tbsp	50	0	0
Strawberry	1 tbsp	50	0	0
Panettone	1 wedge	375	15	36
Panne	1 slice	110	4	32
Phillo dough	1 oz	74	0	0
Pizza bread (1 slice bread, 1 oz cheese)	1 serving	200	10	45
Popovers	1.4 oz	100	4	37
Rolls:				
Butter corn roll	1	200	11	49
Dinner roll	1	120	2	15
French roll	1	140	2	13
Hamburger roll	1	120	2	15
Hard roll	1	140	2	13
Onion roll	1	150	3	18

	AMOUNT	CALORIES	FAT-GRAMS	% FAT
Parkerhouse	1 oz	120	1	7
Soft yeast roll	1	155	7	41
Sourdough roll	1	150	2	12
Vienna roll	1	95	3	28
Scone	1	363	14	33
Sopapilla	1	170	10	33
Spoon bread	2 oz	155	6	35
Sweet breads:				
Apple streusel	1 slice	130	4	28
Banana nut bread	1 slice	165	6	33
Boston brown bread				
(3¼ x ½″)	1 slice	95	1	10
Coffee cake	2½ oz	320	17	48
Cranberry bread	1 slice	95	4	37
Danish krengle	1 sq	230	14	55
Danish pastry				
Fruit	1	235	13	50
Plain	1	220	12	49
Danish twist	1	120	6	45
French crumb				
cake	1 slice	300	16	48
Fruit square	1	250	3	11
Pumpkin bread	1 slice	100	4	37
Sally Lunn	1 slice	240	11	41
Swedish limpa	1 slice	80	1	11
Sweet rolls/buns:				
Butterhorn	1	330	18	49
Caramel bun	1	205	8	35
Caramel nut roll	1	230	11	43
Cinnamon roll	1	290	9	28
Fruit-filled roll	1	220	7	29
Hot cross bun	1	155	4	23
Orange roll	1	195	6	28
Santa Lucia bun	1	205	9	39

	AMOUNT	CALORIES	FAT-GRAMS	% FAT
Sticky bun	1	245	10	37
Sweet potato bun	1	125	1	7
Sweet roll	2½ oz	225	8	32
Tortilla				
Corn (6" diameter)	1	70	1	13
Flour (7" diameter)	1	85	2	21
Waffles				
Round (7" diameter)	1	280	19	61
Square (9")	1	600	40	60

Waffle toppings. *See* Pancakes.

BREAKFAST CEREALS

	AMOUNT	CALORIES	FAT-GRAMS	% FAT
COOKED CEREALS				
Cornmeal mush				
(cornmeal, butter)	1 cup	155	6	35
Cream of rice	¾ cup	110	0	0
Cream of wheat	¾ cup	110	0	0
Farina	⅔ cup	80	0	0
Corn grits	½ cup	55	0	0
Hominy quick grits				
(uncooked)	¼ cup	150	0	0
Oat bran	⅔ cup	110	1	8
Oatmeal	⅔ cup	110	1	8
READY-TO-EAT CEREALS				
All-Bran	⅔ cup	70	1	13
Alpha Bits	1 cup	110	0	0
Boo Berry	1 cup	110	0	0
Bran Flakes	⅔ cup	90	0	0
Cinnamon Toast				
Crunch	1 cup	120	3	22
Cheerios	1¼ cup	110	2	16
Chex	⅔ cup	90	0	0
Cocoa Puffs	1 cup	110	1	8
Corn Flakes	1 cup	100	0	0

	AMOUNT	CALORIES	FAT-GRAMS	% FAT
Frankenberry	1 cup	110	1	8
Froot Loops	1 cup	110	0	0
Frosty Flakes	¾ cup	110	0	0
Fruit & Fibre (dates, raisins, walnuts)	½ cup	90	0	0
Fruity Pebbles	1 cup	120	1	8
Granola	¼ cup	125	4	28
w/ raisins	¼ cup	125	4	29
Grape-Nuts	¼ cup	110	0	0
Flakes	⅞ cup	100	1	9
Honeycomb	1⅓ cup	110	1	8
Lucky Charms	1 cup	110	1	8
Müesli	½ cup	160	3	17
Müeslix Five Grain	½ cup	150	2	12
Nutri-Grain Wheat	⅔ cup	100	0	0
& Raisin	⅔ cup	130	0	0
Oat Bran Flakes	½ cup	100	0	0
Post Toasties	1¼ cup	108	0	0
Product 19	1 cup	100	0	0
Puffed Rice	1 cup	40	0	0
Raisin Bran	¾ cup	120	1	7
Rice Krispies	1 cup	110	0	0
Shredded Wheat	1 biscuit	85	0	0
Bite Size	⅔ cup	110	1	8
Special K	1 cup	110	0	0
Sugar Frosted Flakes	¾ cup	110	0	0
Total	1 cup	110	1	8
Total Corn Flakes	1 cup	110	1	8
Trix	1 cup	110	1	8
Wheaties	1 cup	110	1	8

CHEESE & CHEESE DISHES

	AMOUNT	CALORIES	FAT-GRAMS	% FAT
Asparagus w/ rarebit sauce	6 oz	525	34	58
Cheese:				
American	1 oz	90	7	70
Blue	1 oz	100	9	81
Bonbel	1 oz	100	8	72
Brie	1 oz	95	8	76
Cajun	1 oz	110	9	74
Camembert	1 oz	85	7	74
Cheddar	1 oz	110	9	74
Cream cheese	1 oz	100	10	90
Neufchâtel	1 oz	80	7	79
Whipped	1 oz	100	10	90
Cottage cheese, creamed				
Full-fat	½ cup	120	5	37
Low-fat	½ cup	90	1	10
Edam	1 oz	100	8	72
Feta	1 oz	75	6	72
Gorgonzola	1 oz	100	8	72
Gouda	1 oz	110	9	74
Gruyère	1 oz	120	9	68
Havarti	1 oz	120	11	84

	AMOUNT	CALORIES	FAT-GRAMS	% FAT
Jarlsberg	1 oz	100	7	63
Monterey Jack	1 oz	80	4	45
Mozzarella, low-moisture				
Whole-milk	1 oz	90	7	70
Part-skim	1 oz	80	5	56
Mozzarella, part skim	1 oz	70	5	62
Nacho	1 oz	105	9	76
Parmesan, grated	1 tbsp	25	2	78
Port du Salut	1 oz	100	8	72
Pot cheese	1 oz	109	5	41
Provolone	1 oz	100	7	63
Roquefort	1 oz	105	9	77
String cheese	1 oz	80	5	57
Swiss	1 oz	100	8	72
Taco, shredded	1 oz	100	9	81
Tilsit	1 oz	95	7	66
Cheese blintzes:	3	375	17	40
Cinnamon	3	375	17	40
Crabmeat	3	390	17	39
Pineapple	3	385	17	40
Shrimp	3	390	17	39
Cheese enchilada	1	490	34	62
Cheese fritters	3	365	16	40
Cheese pie	⅛ of 9" pie	330	17	46
Cheese sauce	2 oz	105	8	68
Cheese soup made w/ milk	1 cup	230	15	59
Cheese spaetzle (Austrian)	8 oz	940	51	49
Cheese soufflé	5 oz	325	24	66
Cheese strata	6 oz	315	18	51

	AMOUNT	CALORIES	FAT-GRAMS	% FAT
Chile relleno	1	340	24	64
Emmentaler flan	⅙ of 9" pie	830	58	63
Fondue:				
Fontina (Italian)	6 oz	510	46	81
Swiss fondue (w/ bread)	1 serving	1,515	59	35
Fritelle	6	740	22	27
Paschel pie (cheese, sausage, eggs)	⅙ of 10" pie	1,110	82	66
Polenta cheese torta (Italian)	8 oz	560	28	45
Quiche (⅙ of 9" pie):				
Quiche Jambon Chardonnay	1 slice	1,075	74	62
Quiche Lorraine	1 slice	875	61	63
Quiche Suisse	1 slice	990	72	65
Ricotta quiche	1 slice	925	63	61
Seafood quiche	1 slice	1,005	67	60
Rarebit:				
Asparagus w/ rarebit sauce	6 oz	525	34	58
Bacon rarebit	6 oz	585	41	63
Bacon-tomato rarebit	6 oz	575	39	61
Ham rarebit	6 oz	565	37	59
Onion rarebit (Swiss)	2 slices	945	65	62
Pineapple rarebit	6 oz	525	34	58
Rarebit in oven (Bavarian)	2 slices	620	26	38
Tomato rarebit	6 oz	530	35	59
Welsh rarebit	6 oz	500	34	61

	AMOUNT	CALORIES	FAT-GRAMS	% FAT
Sbrinz casserole (Swiss)	8 oz	305	18	53
Shepherd's Yodel (Bavarian)	2 slices	800	55	62
Swiss bread rosti	6 oz	500	28	50
Swiss ramequin	8 oz	595	31	47
Welsh rarebit	6 oz	500	34	61

DESSERTS & TOPPINGS

DESSERTS	AMOUNT	CALORIES	FAT-GRAMS	% FAT
Almond torte	1/10 of 9" torte	280	20	64
Baklava (2" x 2")	1	430	29	61
Bars:				
Almond toffee bars	2	165	10	54
Chinese chews	2	395	16	37
French lemon bars	2	120	4	29
French nut loaf	1	390	25	57
Fudge nut loaf	1	390	18	41
Hermits	2	275	11	36
Magic Bars	2	205	12	53
Mincemeat strips	2	140	7	45
Orange-date bars	2	205	7	30
Peanut butter crunch	1 pc	235	9	34
Bavarians:				
Banana-lemon	4 oz	160	7	39
Caramel	4 oz	200	11	50
Chocolate	4 oz	245	13	48
Coffee	4 oz	220	15	62
Fruit-nut	4 oz	245	16	59
Orange cream	4 oz	170	7	37

	AMOUNT	CALORIES	FAT-GRAMS	% FAT
Pineapple	4 oz	200	11	49
Raspberry	4 oz	135	7	46
Strawberry	4 oz	150	7	42
Biscuit tortoni	3 oz	345	29	75
Blintzes:				
Cherry	1	385	17	40
Cinnamon cheese	3	375	17	40
Pineapple cheese	3	385	17	40
Brownies:				
Bavarian brownie drop	1	125	8	58
Brownies				
Cake type	2	155	8	47
Chewy type	2	160	9	50
Butterscotch brownies	2	145	7	44
Chocolate coconut brownie	1	345	18	47
Cream cheese brownies	2	390	23	53
Cake:				
Angel food cake	1 slice	145	0	0
w/ icing		220	3	12
Applesauce cake	1 slice	245	9	33
Apricot upside-down cake	1 slice	245	9	33
Baked Alaska	5 oz	390	9	21
Banana cake	1 slice	260	9	31
w/ icing		335	12	32
Black Forest cake				
w/ icing	1 slice	530	20	34
Boston cream pie cake	1/12 of 10" cake	260	8	28
Burnt sugar cake	1 slice	225	9	36
Butter rum pound cake	1/12 of 10" cake	480	19	36

	AMOUNT	CALORIES	FAT-GRAMS	% FAT
Cannoli cake	1/12 of 9" cake	785	35	40
Carrot cake w/ cream cheese icing	1/16 of 10" cake	385	21	49
Carrot spice cake	1 slice	220	10	41
w/ icing		295	13	40
Cheesecake:	1/8 of 9" cake	410	31	68
Chocolate	1/8 of 9" cake	425	29	61
Chocolate hazelnut	1/7 of 7" cake	400	32	72
Chocolate ricotta	1/8 of 8" cake	435	26	53
Peanut butter	1/8 of 9" cake	410	23	50
Pumpkin	1/8 of 9" cake	465	34	66
Strawberry	1/8 of 9" cake	530	31	53
Cherry jubilee cake	1 slice	130	7	49
Chiffon cake	1/12 of 10" cake	230	10	39
w/ icing		305	13	39
Chocolate cake roll	1 slice	360	11	27
w/ icing		465	19	37
Chocolate chiffon cake	1/12 of 10" cake	235	10	38
w/ icing		335	17	45
Chocolate whipped cream cake	1/16 of 10" cake	400	22	49
Christmas fruitcake	1/32 of loaf	275	8	26

	AMOUNT	CALORIES	FAT-GRAMS	% FAT
Devil's food cake	1 slice	190	8	38
w/ icing		295	15	46
Dutch apple cake	1 pc	220	7	29
English plum pudding	1 slice	270	7	23
French crumb cake	1 slice	365	16	39
Fruit coffee cake	1 slice	275	10	33
Fruit pudding cake	2.5 oz	195	7	32
Fruit whipped cream cake	1 slice	305	18	53
German chocolate cake	1 slice	225	12	48
w/ icing		330	19	52
Gingerbread	1 slice	200	8	36
Honeycomb crunch cake	1 slice	405	24	54
Lady Baltimore cake	1 slice	265	11	38
Nut torte	1 slice	195	10	47
Orange coffee cake	1 slice	185	6	29
Peach downside-up cake	1 slice	265	11	37
Peach upside-down cake	1 slice	255	9	32
Peanut butter cake	1 slice	230	10	39
w/ icing		335	13	35
Pineapple upside-down cake	1 slice	255	10	35
Plain cake	1 slice	190	7	33
w/ buttercream icing		265	10	34
w/ chocolate icing		290	14	43
Poor man's cake	1 slice	235	4	15
Pound cake	1/9 of 9" cake	365	21	52

	AMOUNT	CALORIES	FAT-GRAMS	% FAT
Praline cake	1 slice	310	19	55
Prune spice cake	1 slice	200	8	36
Pumpkin cake	1 slice	275	9	30
Sally Lunn	1 slice	240	11	41
Spice cake	1 slice	205	8	35
w/ icing		280	11	36
Sponge cake	1 indiv cake	190	3	14
Sponge roll	1 slice	125	2	14
Swiss nut cake	1 slice	390	24	55
White cake	1 slice	230	9	35
w/ icing		305	12	35
Cannoli	1/11 of 11" shell	530	35	60
Cassata	1 slice	605	19	28
Chocolate éclair (2" x 4")	1	239	13	51
Chocolate pôt de crème	4 oz	315	20	57
Cookies:				
Apricot strips	1	210	9	22
Biscotti (Italian cookies)	1	127	7	50
Brown sugar cookie	1	135	7	47
Butterscotch cookie	1	60	3	45
Cherry Winks	1	95	4	38
Chocolate candy cookie	1	120	4	30
Chocolate-chip cookie	1	105	5	42
Chocolate crumb cookie	1	85	4	42
Chocolate drop cookie	1	165	6	33
Coconut chip cookie	1	135	8	52
Coconut lace cookie	1	45	2	38
Crescent	1	100	7	64
Fortune cookie	1	65	4	55
Ginger cookie	1	165	5	28

	AMOUNT	CALORIES	FAT-GRAMS	% FAT
Ginger crisp	1	60	2	29
Lady finger	1	40	1	20
Lebkuchen	1	55	1	16
Madeleines	2	85	5	53
Meringue cookie	1	35	0	0
Molasses cookie	1	155	7	40
Oatmeal cookie	1	160	7	39
Oatmeal raisin cookie	1	145	7	43
Oatmeal spice cookie	1	110	6	48
Peanut butter candy cookie	1	125	6	43
Peanut butter cookie	1	135	8	54
Peanut butter cup	1	155	9	53
Raisin drop cookie	1	100	4	36
Refrigerator cookie	1	70	3	39
Sandtart	1	80	5	58
Shortbread	1	155	9	52
Snickerdoodle	1	80	3	35
Spritz	1	70	4	50
Sugar cookie	1	150	6	36
Sugar plum cookie	1	45	2	40
Swedish ginger cookie	1	40	2	43
Turtle cookies	2	195	10	46
Vanilla butter cookies	2	65	3	42
Cream puff w/ custard filling (3½" x 2")	1	303	18	54
Crepes:				
Crepes suzette	3	600	31	46
Dessert crepe (unfilled)	1	135	7	47
Raspberry crepes	2	540	21	35
Custards:				
Burnt cream	4 oz	325	25	69
Caramel flan	¾ cup	230	6	23

	AMOUNT	CALORIES	FAT-GRAMS	% FAT
Crème brulée	4 oz	325	25	69
Custard	4 oz	160	5	28
Spanish cream	4 oz	185	9	44
English trifle	4 oz	465	23	44
Frozen yogurt, soft-serve, average	½ cup	120	5	38
Low-fat, average	½ cup	100	2	18
Nonfat, average	½ cup	110	0	0
Fruit:				
Apples				
Applesauce	1 cup	190	1	5
Baked apple	1	185	1	5
Baked date-nut apple	1	290	7	22
Caramel apple	1	430	20	42
Caramel fried apples	⅓ apple	205	5	22
Taffy apple	1	390	11	25
Apricot tart	⅛ of 10" pie	470	13	25
Apricots, stewed	6 halves	60	0	0
Banana dessert fritters	2	310	5	14
Cherries Jubilee (sauce only)	4 oz	65	0	0
Cherry blintz	1	385	17	40
Fruit & 2 oz cheese	1 serving	310	18	52
Fruit compote	1 serving	90	0	0
Fruit cup	½ cup	55	0	0
Fruit-nut Bavarian	4 oz	245	16	59
Fruit plate (fruit only)	1 serving	80	0	0
Italian cream w/ raspberries	1 serving	265	16	55
Peaches flambé	4 oz	420	17	36

	AMOUNT	CALORIES	FAT-GRAMS	% FAT
Pineapple cheese blintz	3	385	17	40
Poached pear w/ raspberry sauce	1 pear	490	12	22
Prunes, stewed	3 prunes	85	0	0
Prune whip	2 oz	130	1	7
Strawberries Romanoff	4 oz	115	4	31
Ice cream:				
Fat-free, average	½ cup	90	0	0
Sealtest Black Cherry	½ cup	100	0	0
Simple Pleasures Chocolate	½ cup	130	0	0
Premium (10% fat), average	½ cup	135	7	47
Borden Chocolate	½ cup	160	10	56
Breyers Strawberry	½ cup	130	6	42
Dreyer's Vanilla	½ cup	160	10	56
Super premium (16% fat), average	½ cup	175	12	62
Ben & Jerry's Chocolate	½ cup	290	18	56
Häagen-Dazs Strawberry	½ cup	250	15	54
Vanilla	½ cup	260	17	57
Ice cream, soft-serve	½ cup	200	12	54
Ice cream bar, chocolate-coated:				
Premium, average	1	180	12	60
Dolly Madison	1	200	12	54
Klondike	1	290	20	62

	AMOUNT	CALORIES	FAT-GRAMS	% FAT
Super premium,				
average	1	340	22	58
Dove Bar	1	350	22	57
Häagen-Dazs	1	390	27	62
Ice cream bombe	1	270	14	47
Ice cream cake				
(2 oz ice cream,				
2 oz sauce):				
Butterscotch	1 slice	355	14	35
Chocolate	1 slice	385	15	38
Ice cream cake roll	1 slice	160	7	39
Ice cream cone:				
Chocolate	1 scoop	180	10	50
	2 scoops	360	20	50
Vanilla	1 scoop	170	8	42
	2 scoops	320	16	45
Cone only				
Comet	1	40	0	0
Sugar	1	55	1	16
Waffle				
Small	1	60	1	15
Large	1	200	3	14
Ice cream drumstick	1 sm	190	10	48
	1 lg	350	19	49
Ice cream pie				
(⅛ of 10″ pie):				
Chocolate	1 slice	680	27	36
Pralines 'n				
Cream	1 slice	810	46	51
Ice cream puff	1	225	7	28
Ice cream sandwich,				
average:	1	170	6	32
Eskimo Pie, Original	1	140	10	64
Good Humor	1	160	5	28

	AMOUNT	CALORIES	FAT-GRAMS	% FAT
Ice cream sundaes:				
Banana split (3 scoops ice cream w/ sauce, whipped cream, nuts, cherry)	1	1,350	76	51
Eskimo Boat	1	705	9	11
Two-scoop sundae:				
w/ butterscotch topping	1	535	25	42
w/ hot fudge	1	540	25	42
Chocolate ice cream, chocolate sauce, whipped cream, cherry)	1	1,145	61	47
Vanilla ice cream, chocolate sauce, whipped cream, cherry)	1	1,085	61	50
Vanilla ice cream, strawberry syrup, whipped cream, nuts, cherry	1	1,065	57	48
Ice cream torte	4 oz	395	22	50
Ice milk (1% fat), average:	½ cup	90	3	30
Carnation Chocolate	½ cup	90	2	20
Borden Strawberry	½ cup	90	2	20
Weight Watchers Vanilla	½ cup	100	3	27
Ice milk, soft-serve, average	½ cup	175	2	16

	AMOUNT	CALORIES	FAT-GRAMS	% FAT
Ices:				
Italian ice	6 oz	140	0	0
Lemon ice	6 oz	140	0	0
Watermelon ice	6 oz	140	0	0
Mousse:				
Apricot	6 oz	360	3	7
Chocolate	1 cup	380	31	73
Peach chiffon	4 oz	200	5	22
Parisian cheese torte	1 slice	270	17	57
Pavlova	⅛ of 9″ cake	220	11	45
Pie:				
Apple Betty	4 oz	215	5	21
Apple crisp	4 oz	220	4	16
w/ cheese (6″ x 8″)	1 serving	260	11	38
Apple dumplings	1 apple	505	24	43
Apple streusel	4 oz	270	10	33
Apricot crunch (6″ x 8″)	1 serving	315	16	45
Black bottom pie	⅛ of 10″ pie	380	16	38
Brown sugar pie	⅛ of 10″ pie	585	25	38
Chiffon pie (⅛ of 10″ pie):				
Banana	1 slice	555	37	60
Chocolate	1 slice	595	41	62
Egg Nog	1 slice	655	40	55
Lime	1 slice	600	38	57
Mocha	1 slice	610	41	60
Orange	1 slice	605	38	57
Peach	1 slice	580	38	59
Peanut crunch	1 slice	700	42	54

	AMOUNT	CALORIES	FAT-GRAMS	% FAT
Peppermint	1 slice	680	40	53
Pineapple	1 slice	580	38	59
Pumpkin	1 slice	665	38	51
Strawberry	1 slice	585	38	58
Chocolate pecan pie	1 slice	600	31	46
Chocolate silk pie	1 slice	600	40	60
Cobbler:				
Apple	5 oz	225	4	16
Blueberry	5 oz	250	4	14
Cherry	5 oz	260	4	14
Peach	5 oz	165	4	22
Pineapple-apricot	4 oz	220	4	16
Purple plum	5 oz	195	4	18
Coconut custard pie	⅛ of 10″ pie	365	18	45
Coconut macaroon pie	⅛ of 10″ pie	635	36	51
Cranberry crunch (6″ x 8″)	1 serving	470	21	40
Cream cheese pie	1 slice	385	25	58
Cream pie (⅛ of 10″ pie):	1 slice	435	30	62
Banana	1 slice	445	30	60
Bavarian	1 slice	315	17	49
Butterscotch	1 slice	400	20	45
Chocolate	1 slice	465	23	45
Coconut	1 slice	470	32	61
Date	1 slice	475	30	57
Raisin	1 slice	710	43	54
Crustless coconut pie	1 slice	380	18	42
Custard pie	1 slice	325	16	44
Date crunch (6″ x 8″)	1 serving	425	17	36

	AMOUNT	CALORIES	FAT-GRAMS	% FAT
Fruit pie				
(⅛ of 10″ pie):				
Apple	1 slice	495	20	36
Apricot	1 slice	455	20	40
Blackberry	1 slice	440	20	41
Blueberry	1 slice	435	20	41
Cherry	1 slice	465	20	39
Cherry glaze	1 slice	425	15	32
Peach	1 slice	480	20	37
Pineapple	1 slice	630	31	44
Strawberry	1 slice	440	20	41
Strawberry parfait	1 slice	630	39	56
Strawberry rhubarb	1 slice	415	19	41
French silk pie. *See* Chocolate silk pie.				
Grasshopper pie	⅙ of 9″ pie	575	35	55
Key lime pie	⅙ of 9″ pie	460	19	37
Lemon chess pie	⅛ of 10″ pie	600	23	35
Lemon meringue pie	⅛ of 10″ pie	655	35	48
Lemon sponge chess pie	⅛ of 10″ pie	665	35	47
Mincemeat pie	⅛ of 10″ pie	510	20	35
Mud pie	⅛ of 10″ pie	610	41	60
Peach crisp	4 oz	235	9	34
Peanut butter pie	⅛ of 10″ pie	675	40	55
Pear crisp	4 oz	180	6	30

	AMOUNT	CALORIES	FAT-GRAMS	% FAT
Pecan pie	1/8 of 10" pie	800	43	48
Pumpkin pie	1/8 of 10" pie	520	31	54
Raisin pie	1/8 of 10" pie	480	20	37
Rhubarb crisp	1/2 cup	185	4	19
Shoofly pie	1/8 of 10" pie	705	38	49
Southern-style lemon icebox pie	1/8 of 10" pie	765	29	34
Pudding:				
Banana meringue	4 oz	195	7	32
Blueberry crumb	1 sq	295	14	43
Bread	4 oz	175	5	26
Coconut	4 oz	185	7	34
Orange	4 oz	155	5	29
Brownie rice	4 oz	240	9	34
Butterscotch	4 oz	225	9	36
Caramel cake (4" x 6")	1 serving	315	11	31
Caramel raisin	4 oz	320	5	14
Chocolate	4 oz	185	6	29
Chocolate fudge	4 oz	370	10	24
Coconut	4 oz	235	8	31
Floating Island	4 oz	185	6	29
Fruit	4 oz	225	7	28
Baked	4 oz	360	18	45
Hunter	4 oz	325	16	44
Indian	4 oz	220	8	33
Lemon sponge	4 oz	220	10	41
Marble cake	1 slice	160	11	61
Orange meringue	4 oz	210	3	13

	AMOUNT	CALORIES	FAT-GRAMS	% FAT
Pear	4 oz	110	1	8
Pineapple Danish	4 oz	215	6	25
Pompadour	5 oz	280	9	29
Rice	4 oz	180	4	20
Baked	½ cup	240	7	26
Rice nut	4 oz	230	10	39
Tapioca	4 oz	150	4	24
Torte	4 oz	180	6	30
Vanilla	4 oz	265	8	27
Ricotta-strawberry manicotti w/ chocolate topping	1 shell	325	17	47
Shortcake:				
Peach shortcake	1 serving	425	20	42
Shortcake biscuit w/ fruit (3 oz biscuit, 2 oz fruit, 1 oz cream)	1 serving	270	17	57
Sorbet & ice cream, average:	½ cup	190	8	38
Orange sorbet & vanilla ice cream	½ cup	190	8	38
Raspberry sorbet & vanilla ice cream	½ cup	180	7	35
Soufflé:				
Chocolate	4 oz	230	13	51
Coconut	4 oz	175	9	47
Orange	4 oz	155	8	46
Tiramisu	⅟₇ of 9″ cake	255	17	60
Vanilla cream square	1	90	5	50
White chocolate-hazelnut tartufo	1	540	38	63
Zabaglione	4 oz	120	4	30

	AMOUNT	CALORIES	FAT-GRAMS	% FAT

NONDAIRY DESSERTS

	AMOUNT	CALORIES	FAT-GRAMS	% FAT
Ice cream, average	½ cup	150	8	48
Mocha mix				
Chocolate	½ cup	160	10	56
Strawberry	½ cup	140	7	45
Tofutti vanilla	½ cup	200	11	50
Light	½ cup	90	0	0
Soft-serve, vanilla	½ cup	160	8	45
Light	½ cup	90	1	10
Frozen fruit bar, average:	1	80	0	0
Dole Cherry Bar	1	70	0	0
Minute Maid Grape Bar	1	60	0	0
Sunkist Orange Bar	1	70	0	0
Sherbet, average	½ cup	110	1	8
Borden Lemon	½ cup	110	1	8
Borden Orange	½ cup	110	1	8
Sorbet, average	½ cup	120	0	0
Dole Mandarin Orange	½ cup	110	0	0
Dole Peach	½ cup	120	0	0

TOPPINGS

	AMOUNT	CALORIES	FAT-GRAMS	% FAT
Blueberries, fresh	2 tbsp	10	0	0
Blueberry sauce	2 tbsp	50	0	0
Butterfinger, crumbled	2 tbsp	130	5	35
Butterscotch topping	2 tbsp	140	1	6
Caramel topping	2 tbsp	140	1	6
Cherry topping	2 tbsp	100	0	0
Chocolate-chip cookie, crumbled	2 tbsp	130	6	42

	AMOUNT	CALORIES	FAT-GRAMS	% FAT
Chocolate fudge topping	2 tbsp	125	5	36
Chocolate topping	2 tbsp	90	1	10
Coconut, shredded	2 tbsp	60	4	60
Fruit cocktail, juice-pack, canned	2 tbsp	15	0	0
Granola	2 tbsp	70	4	13
Hard sauce	2 tbsp	140	6	39
Heath bar, crumbled	2 tbsp	145	9	56
Hot fudge	2 tbsp	110	4	33
Lemon sauce	2 tbsp	60	2	30
M&M's:				
Plain	2 tbsp	135	6	40
Peanut	2 tbsp	150	7	42
Maraschino cherry	1	10	0	0
Marshmallow	2 tbsp	120	0	0
Mixed nuts	2 tbsp	170	15	79
Nut topping	1 oz	180	16	80
Oreo cookies, crumbled	2 tbsp	140	6	39
Peanut butter caramel	2 tbsp	150	2	12
Peanuts	2 tbsp	165	14	76
Pecans in syrup	2 tbsp	130	1	7
Pineapple topping	2 tbsp	100	0	0
Raisins:	2 tbsp	55	0	0
Chocolate-covered	2 tbsp	120	5	38
Yogurt-covered	2 tbsp	135	6	40
Red raspberry topping	1 tbsp	50	0	0
Reese's Pieces	2 tbsp	140	6	39
Sprinkles, chocolate	1 tbsp	30	0	0
Strawberries, fresh	2 tbsp	5	0	0
Strawberry topping	2 tbsp	120	0	0

	AMOUNT	CALORIES	FAT-GRAMS	% FAT
Walnuts in syrup	2 tbsp	130	1	7
Walnut topping	1 tbsp	90	5	50
Whipped toppings:				
Almond whipped cream	½ cup	175	17	88
Almond whipped topping	½ cup	90	5	49
Nondairy whipped topping	½ cup	95	8	76
Pressurized whipped cream	½ cup	75	7	84
Whipped cream, fresh	½ cup	205	22	96

EGGS & EGG DISHES

	AMOUNT	CALORIES	FAT-GRAMS	% FAT
Baked (shirred) eggs				
w/ cheese	2 eggs	265	22	74
Boiled egg	1	75	5	41
Breakfast pizza (eggs, olives, mushrooms, tomato)	⅙ of 12″ pie	325	21	58
Calf brains & eggs	8 oz	690	57	75
Cheesy egg roll-up on tortilla	1	395	24	55
Chili relleno	1	340	24	64
Curried eggs	5 oz	305	17	50
Deviled eggs	2 halves	145	13	80
Egg blintzes	2	186	6	29
Egg foo yong (2-oz patties)	2 patties	210	15	65
Egg substitute (Egg Beaters)	¼ cup	25	0	0
w/ cheese		130	6	41
Egg salad	½ cup	310	28	81
Egg turnover w/ 2 oz cheese sauce	1 serving	470	34	65

	AMOUNT	CALORIES	FAT-GRAMS	% FAT
Eggs à la goldenrod (eggs, toast, cream sauce)	5 oz	810	52	58
Eggs à la king	5 oz	690	43	56
Eggs à la Purgatory	2 eggs	220	14	57
Eggs w/ avocado sauce	2 eggs	400	33	74
Eggs Benedict (½ English muffin, 1 egg, ham, sauce)	1 serving	410	32	70
Eggs Benedict casserole	1 serving	395	28	64
Eggs w/ black beans & plantains	2 eggs	400	33	74
Eggs in cheese sauce	6 oz	355	22	56
Eggs on English muffin	2 eggs	280	17	55
Eggs Florentine	2 tarts	530	40	68
Eggs Park Avenue (eggs, lox, sour cream, cream cheese, Hollandaise sauce)	6 oz	935	92	88
Eggs Romano (2 eggs, spinach, olives, Romano)	1 serving	375	25	60
Eggs in shirts	3 eggs	440	40	82
Eggs Sojourn (2 eggs, crab & shrimp meat, English muffin, Hollandaise sauce)	1 serving	1,790	159	80
Egg on tortilla (1 egg, 1 corn tortilla, cheese, salsa)	1 serving	345	25	65
Fried egg	1	105	8	69

	AMOUNT	CALORIES	FAT-GRAMS	% FAT
Frittata				
w/ mushrooms	3 eggs	310	23	67
w/ zucchini, cheese & artichokes	3 eggs	585	47	72
Huevos con queso in tortilla (2 eggs, cheese, tortilla sauce)	1 serving	745	53	64
Huevos leone (bacon omelet w/ tortilla)	10 oz	565	42	67
Huevos rancheros	6 oz	390	25	58
Hungarian gulyas (egg, yogurt, ham, cheese, sunflower seeds)	5 oz	425	34	72
Oeufs Antoine (eggs, bacon, capers, English muffin, Mornay sauce)	6 oz	705	50	64
Omelets (3 eggs):				
Bacon omelet	1	375	28	67
Basque omelet (w/ peppers, onion, tomato)	1	430	36	75
Cheese omelet	1	355	26	66
Farmer-style omelet (eggs, onion, ham, potatoes)	1	405	30	67
Ham omelet	1	330	23	63
Herb omelet	1	295	21	64
Mushroom omelet	1	300	22	66
Plain omelet	1	330	21	57

	AMOUNT	CALORIES	FAT-GRAMS	% FAT
Spanish omelet (w/ Creole sauce)	1	350	25	64
Western omelet (eggs, bacon, ham, onion, peppers)	1	355	25	63
Poached egg:	1	75	5	41
Creamy poached egg (1 egg on ½ English muffin w/ cheese sauce)	1 serving	325	20	56
Poached eggs Henri (eggs, toast, Canadian bacon, asparagus, Hollandaise sauce)	6 oz	690	55	72
Scrambled eggs (2 large eggs):	4 oz	200	16	72
w/ ham	4 oz	275	21	68
w/ herbs	4 oz	205	15	66
w/ mushrooms	4 oz	210	15	64
w/ smoked salmon	4 oz	305	19	56
Soufflé:				
Cheese	6 oz	325	24	66
Spinach	6 oz	320	18	51
Swiss eggs (eggs, Swiss cheese, Gruyère)	3 eggs	505	44	78
Zucchini & egg crepes	2 crepes	445	29	58

GARNISHES & ENTRÉE ACCOMPANI-MENTS

	AMOUNT	CALORIES	FAT-GRAMS	% FAT
Apples:				
Apple fritter rings	3 fritters	340	14	37
Caramel apples	4 oz	150	4	24
Cinnamon apple ring	1 serving	50	1	21
Escalloped apples	4 oz	180	6	30
French apple puffs	2	260	15	52
Glazed apples	2 slices	175	6	31
Bananas, fried	2 halves	205	12	53
Blueberry sinkers	2	260	14	48
Fritters:				
Apple fritter rings	3 fritters	340	14	37
Cherry fritters	2	260	15	52
Royal Hawaiian fritters	2	265	15	51
Glazed peach	½ peach	130	2	14
Spiced fruit	1 serving	110	0	0
Yorkshire pudding (3" square)	1 serving	171	10	52

MEATS & MEAT DISHES

BEEF	AMOUNT	CALORIES	FAT-GRAMS	% FAT
Beef & green bean casserole	8 oz	245	14	51
Beef, biscuit & gravy	1 serving	480	31	58
Beef Burgundy	6 oz	300	10	30
Beef Creole	6 oz	285	9	28
Beef curry	6 oz	275	9	29
Beef goulash	6 oz	300	11	33
Beef kabob teriyaki	1 kabob	380	14	33
Beef noodle casserole	8 oz	420	19	40
Beef paprikash	6 oz	340	15	40
Beef pot pie	8 oz	840	62	66
Beef roulade w/ 2 oz sauce	1 serving	460	24	47
Beef Stroganoff	6 oz	340	20	53
Beef turnover	1	565	42	67
Beef Wellington	4 oz	485	30	55
Beef w/ oyster sauce	6 oz	270	16	54
Braised beef w/ gravy (6 oz meat, 2.5 oz gravy)	1 serving	565	28	44
Brisket of beef	4 oz	480	25	47

	AMOUNT	CALORIES	FAT-GRAMS	% FAT
Chicken-fried steak	4 oz	580	41	64
Chili:				
Chili con carne	8 oz	205	6	26
Chili Santa Fe	10 oz	340	17	45
Chili verde	8 oz	270	15	50
Chili w/ macaroni	8 oz	255	6	21
Chipped beef:				
Chipped beef w/ egg	6 oz	235	15	57
Chipped beef				
w/ macaroni	8 oz	315	17	48
Creamed chipped				
beef	6 oz	300	20	60
Corned beef	2.5 oz	215	11	46
Golabki (cabbage roll)	1	260	13	45
Hamburger patty	4 oz	275	19	62
Hamburger pie	8 oz	475	28	53
Hash:				
Beef	8 oz	390	23	53
Corned beef	8 oz	320	17	48
Red flannel	8 oz	425	22	46
Liver, sautéed	3.5 oz	315	20	57
Macaroni, beef &				
tomato casserole	8 oz	285	13	41
Meatballs:				
Italian meatballs	3.5 oz	310	19	55
Meatballs in sour				
cream gravy				
(1″ meatballs,	3			
1.5 oz gravy)	meatballs	370	26	63
Meatballs Stroganoff				
(1″ meatballs,	3			
2 oz sauce)	meatballs	370	23	56
Porcupine meatballs				
(1″ each)	3	275	14	46

	AMOUNT	CALORIES	FAT-GRAMS	% FAT
Swedish meatballs (1" meatballs, sauce)	3 meatballs	285	16	50
Meat loaf	4 oz	295	17	52
Mexican-style beef:				
Burrito	1	390	14	32
w/ sour cream		440	20	41
Carne Asada	6 oz	365	25	61
Carnitas de Res (sirloin strips, vegetables, sauce)	6 oz	305	16	47
Chimichanga (beef, cheese, tortilla, sour cream)	1	660	44	60
Enchilada w/ sour cream	1	435	30	62
Fajita (beef, peppers, onion, tortilla)	1	510	30	53
w/ 2 tbsp guacamole & 2 tbsp sour cream		615	40	59
Flauta (6" tortilla, beef filling)	1	255	15	53
w/ 2 tbsp guacamole & 2 tbsp sour cream		355	25	63
Quesadilla (6")	1	430	26	54
Short ribs chipotle sauce	1 meaty rib	580	25	39
Sopito	1	490	29	53

	AMOUNT	CALORIES	FAT-GRAMS	% FAT
Taco (1 corn tortilla, ⅓ cup filling)	1	280	16	51
w/ 2 tbsp guacamole & 2 tbsp sour cream		385	26	61
Tamale pie	8 oz	310	13	38
Tamales (2 small w/ sauce)	1 serving	345	20	52
Tostada (beef, beans, cheese, olives, avocado, sour cream) (8″)	1	1,005	64	57
Oriental-style beef:				
Bahmi Goreng w/ sauce (beef, noodles, vegetables)	main dish	465	16	31
per 1 tbsp peanut sauce	*add*	40	3	68
Cashew beef	main dish	670	44	59
Chinese beef & green pepper stir-fry	6 oz	295	11	34
Ginger beef stir-fry	6 oz	305	10	29
Mongolian beef (w/ green onions, rice noodles)	main dish	480	22	41
Noodles & beef w/ black bean sauce	main dish	680	36	48
Oyster sauce beef	6 oz	270	16	54
Peking beef	main dish	435	29	60

	AMOUNT	CALORIES	FAT-GRAMS	% FAT
Stir-fried beef (w/ peppers, onions, mushrooms, snow peas)	7 oz	345	22	57
w/ bok choy	main dish	405	26	57
w/ broccoli	7 oz	320	19	54
w/ napa cabbage	main dish	385	23	54
w/ oyster sauce over noodles	8 oz	435	20	41
w/ snow peas & water chestnuts	8 oz	435	29	60
Szechuan beef	7 oz	350	17	44
Ragout of beef	main dish	640	29	40
Roasts:				
Pot roast (2.5 oz beef, 2 oz gravy)	1 serving	245	12	44
Prime rib roast (lean only)	8 oz	405	23	51
Prime rib roast, blackened	8 oz	585	44	68
Roast boneless rib of beef	8 oz	405	23	50
Roast tenderloin of beef	3 oz	155	7	40
Standing rib roast	8 oz	405	23	51
Sauerbraten (4 oz meat, 4 oz gravy)	1 serving	590	36	55
Short ribs:				
Barbecued	1 rib	560	48	85
Braised	1 rib	590	51	77
Steaks:				
Bavarian beef steak	4 oz	285	16	51
Beef steak teriyaki	4 oz	310	15	44

	AMOUNT	CALORIES	FAT-GRAMS	% FAT
Beef tips & eggplant				
w/ tomato sauce	4 oz	400	16	36
Braised beef steak	4 oz	230	11	43
w/ onions	4 oz	275	13	43
Braised cubed beef	6 oz	275	9	30
Chopped sirloin steak	5 oz	225	9	36
Delmonico steak				
(choice)				
Lean & fat	8 oz	570	44	70
Lean only	8 oz	370	20	49
Filet mignon (prime)				
Lean & fat	8 oz	450	37	74
Lean only	8 oz	385	20	47
London broil	5 oz	300	22	66
New York steak,				
lean only	8 oz	385	20	47
Pepper steak	5 oz	245	15	55
Porterhouse steak				
(choice)				
Lean & fat	8 oz	650	52	72
Lean only	8 oz	360	18	45
Rib-eye steak				
(choice)				
Lean & fat	8 oz	570	44	70
Lean only	8 oz	370	20	49
Round steak Italienne	4 oz	210	9	38
Salisbury steak	5 oz	335	20	53
w/ tomato sauce		355	22	56
Sirloin steak (prime)				
Lean & fat	8 oz	655	27	37
Lean only	8 oz	310	12	35
w/ Béarnaise				
sauce, mushrooms				
& truffles	6 oz	805	61	68

MEATS / MEAT DISHES

	AMOUNT	CALORIES	FAT-GRAMS	% FAT
w/ escargots (broiled beef loin steak), escargots	1 steak	675	41	55
Skirt steak (lean only)	6 oz	385	22	51
Spanish-style steak (w/ Creole sauce)	4 oz	245	11	40
Steak au poivre	10 oz	670	38	51
Steak Barrington (bacon-wrapped broiled ground round)	8 oz	510	35	62
Steak Oscar	6 oz	805	61	68
Steak teriyaki	4 oz	325	15	41
Stuffed flank steak	5 oz	330	19	52
Swiss steak	4 oz	250	13	47
w/ gravy	4 oz	300	18	54
w/ sour cream	5 oz	260	22	77
T-bone steak (choice)				
Lean & fat	8 oz	735	55	68
Lean only	8 oz	485	23	43
Tenderloin (prime)				
Lean & fat	5.5 oz	450	37	74
Lean only	8 oz	385	20	47
Tenderloin tips (on toast points, w/ mushrooms, Burgundy sauce)	5 oz	485	28	52
Top loin steak (prime)				
Lean & fat	10 oz	805	63	71
Lean only	8 oz	425	24	51

	AMOUNT	CALORIES	FAT-GRAMS	% FAT
Tournedos à la crème (beef tournedo, cream sauce)	8 oz	635	43	61
Tournedos Messina (beef fillet, bread, chicken liver pâté, artichokes, mushrooms)	8 oz	730	49	60
Stews:				
Beef stew	8 oz	315	12	35
Beef stew Bordelaise	8 oz	375	17	40
Irish stew	8 oz	280	7	22
Old-fashioned beef stew w/ dumplings	8 oz	745	30	36
Stuffed cabbage	1 cabbage	330	20	54
Stuffed pepper	½ pepper	320	20	56
w/ cheese		525	30	51
Tomato beef	main dish	310	18	52
Tongue, smoked	2.5 oz	260	19	65

GAME

	AMOUNT	CALORIES	FAT-GRAMS	% FAT
Stewed rabbit	¼ rabbit	380	16	38
Venison chop, marinated	1	315	12	34
Venison pot roast	4 oz	330	12	33
Venison sauerbraten	4 oz	235	9	34

LAMB

	AMOUNT	CALORIES	FAT-GRAMS	% FAT
BBQ lamb ribs	1	265	11	37
Boiled lamb w/ dill sauce	6 oz	300	15	45
Braised lamb shank	1	515	33	58
Braised lamb shoulder chop	1	275	14	46

	AMOUNT	CALORIES	FAT-GRAMS	% FAT
Carbonnade of lamb	6 oz	290	13	40
Chili:				
Chili Santa Fe	8 oz	345	17	44
New Mexican green chili	8 oz	340	16	43
Crown roast of lamb w/ stuffing	2 chops	745	34	91
Greek-style lamb w/ orzo (4 oz meat, 2 oz orzo)	1 serving	415	12	26
Hunter-style lamb (w/ garlic, rosemary)	7 oz	495	41	75
Lamb & artichoke w/ avgolemono sauce (1 lamb shank, 3 oz vegetable, sauce)	1 serving	310	11	32
Lamb & couscous	6 oz	345	14	36
Lamb curry	6 oz	325	18	50
Lamb fricassee	6 oz	265	10	34
Lamb patty	4 oz	235	15	57
Lamb pilaf	6 oz	375	13	31
Lamb pot pie	8 oz	370	19	46
Lamb riblets	2	390	18	41
Lamb Salonika (w/ mushrooms & cream sauce)	6 oz	280	18	58
Lamb scallops À la crème (lamb leg, mushrooms, onions, cream sauce)	6 oz	260	16	56

	AMOUNT	CALORIES	FAT GRAMS	% FAT
Provençal (lamb leg, onion, garlic, wine, tomatoes)	6 oz	285	12	38
Lamb stew	6 oz	310	21	61
Leg of lamb:				
Leg of lamb roast	3 oz	180	7	35
w/ potatoes & vegetables	6 oz	455	16	32
Stuffed leg of lamb, en croûte	6 oz	665	36	49
Moussaka	8 oz	685	33	43
Navarin of spring lamb	6 oz	485	28	52
New Mexican green chili	8 oz	340	16	43
Rack of lamb	4 oz	470	34	65
Roast lamb shoulder	6 oz	250	16	57
Stuffed	6 oz	680	34	45
Rolled braised lamb shoulder	6 oz	645	36	50
Russian bitki lamb patties	4 oz	515	36	63
Shepherd's pie	10 oz	330	12	33
Shish kabob	1 kabob	305	16	48
Stuffed breast of lamb	6 oz	335	13	35
Stuffed Turks (½ stuffed green pepper)	1 serving	255	13	46

PORK

	AMOUNT	CALORIES	FAT GRAMS	% FAT
Bacon				
Medium slice	0.3 oz	50	4	79
Thick slice	0.4 oz	70	6	79
Thin slice	0.1 oz	15	1	79
Canadian bacon	2 slices	85	4	42

	AMOUNT	CALORIES	FAT-GRAMS	% FAT
Ham:				
Baked ham	2.5 oz	155	8	46
Creamed ham	6 oz	285	18	56
Escalloped ham & cabbage (w/ creamy cheese sauce)	8 oz	390	23	53
Escalloped ham & macaroni (w/ cheese sauce)	8 oz	420	21	45
Ham à la king (w/ mushrooms, cream sauce)	6 oz	270	16	53
Ham & lima beans	8 oz	280	6	19
Ham & noodles au gratin	8 oz	465	27	52
Ham & potatoes au gratin	8 oz	400	22	49
Ham & sweet potatoes w/ apples	8 oz	345	7	18
Ham crepes w/ 2 oz sauce	2 crepes	400	16	36
Ham, macaroni & tomato casserole	8 oz	255	9	10
Ham patty	5 oz raw	305	14	41
Ham roll au gratin (ham, broccoli, toast, sauce)	main dish	670	39	52
Ham shortcake (ham, corn bread, sauce)	8 oz	355	15	38
Ham steak, grilled	3 oz	180	9	45

	AMOUNT	CALORIES	FAT-GRAMS	% FAT
Honey glazed ham steak, baked	3 oz	240	10	37
Roast fresh ham	2.5 oz	105	5	42
Cashew pork & pea pods	main dish	555	21	34
Fish-flavored pork	main dish	435	24	50
Hungarian pork goulash	8 oz	295	19	58
Moo goo gai pan	main dish	545	15	25
Moo shu pork	main dish	630	38	54
Mexicali pork chili	8 oz	590	41	63
Noodles w/ pork & peanut sauce	main dish	580	25	39
Polsa (Swedish hash)	10 oz	200	7	32
Pork & Spanish rice	8 oz	335	13	35
Pork burrito	1	385	24	56
w/ sour cream		435	30	62
Pork chimichanga (pork, cheese, tortilla, sour cream)	1	665	44	60
Pork chops:				
BBQ	1 chop	390	25	57
Beer-braised, w/ brown sauce	1 chop	655	45	62
Breaded	1 chop	310	13	38
Creole-style	1 chop	335	25	67
in orange sauce	1 chop	415	30	65
Italian-style, w/ fried potatoes	1 serving	595	28	43
Smoked	1 chop	290	11	34
Stuffed (bread dressing)	1 chop	490	36	66
w/ Madeira sauce	1 chop	505	31	55
Pork chop suey	8 oz	195	10	46

	AMOUNT	CALORIES	FAT-GRAMS	% FAT
Pork chow mein	6 oz	270	18	59
Pork cutlet, breaded	1	260	10	35
Pork fried rice	1 cup	355	17	43
Pork kabob	1	345	12	31
Pork loaf	4 oz	285	13	41
Pork meatballs				
w/ ginger glaze	6 sm	235	9	35
Pork, noodle & cheese				
casserole	8 oz	390	20	46
Pork ragout	8 oz	600	25	37
Pork, shrimp,				
vegetables & rice				
(Thai-style)	main dish	565	30	48
Pork stew	8 oz	600	25	37
Pork taco				
(1 corn tortilla,				
⅓ cup filling)	1	280	16	51
w/ 2 tbsp sour				
cream		335	22	59
w/ 2 tbsp sour				
cream & 2 tbsp				
guacamole		385	26	61
Pork tenderloin				
in mushroom cream				
sauce	4 oz	260	14	48
Oriental	6 oz	285	16	57
w/ apple-celery				
dressing	main dish	345	18	47
w/ peppers				
& onions	4 oz	280	13	42
Pork Tetrazzini	1 cup	345	20	52
Roast loin of pork,				
bone in	4 oz	275	16	52
Roast suckling pig	6 oz	410	21	46

	AMOUNT	CALORIES	FAT-GRAMS	% FAT
Sausages:				
Bockwurst	4 oz	260	24	83
Bratwurst	4 oz	340	28	74
Chorizo (Mexican sausage)	4 oz	300	24	71
Italian sausage	4 oz	265	24	82
w/ green peppers		295	24	76
Italian sausage, braised, w/ polenta	1 sausage	505	30	53
Knockwurst (pork & beef)	3.5 oz	280	15	48
Polish sausage, fresh	4 oz	230	20	78
Sausage links (1 oz each)	1	110	11	90
Sausage patty	3 oz	330	33	90
Scallopini à la Marsala	1 cutlet	300	18	54
Scrapple (2 slices)	3 oz	255	8	28
Spareribs:				
BBQ spareribs	8 oz	645	43	60
Hawaiian spareribs	8 oz	600	43	64
Spareribs & sauerkraut (8 oz ribs, 4 oz sauerkraut)	1 serving	595	43	65
Stir-fried pork w/ vegetables	main dish	435	24	50
Swedish meatballs (1″ each)	6	585	37	57
Sweet & sour pork	8 oz	255	8	28
Sweet & sour pork balls (1″ each)	3	225	7	28
Szechuan pork	main dish	300	20	60
Twice-cooked pork	main dish	300	20	60

VEAL

	AMOUNT	CALORIES	FAT-GRAMS	% FAT
Braised veal shank w/ risotto	1 shank	495	11	20
Braised veal w/ prosciutto & escarole	7 oz	360	18	45
Breaded veal cutlet	4 oz	385	15	35
Calf's liver	6 oz	445	33	68
Hungarian veal paprikash (veal, onions, cream sauce)	6 oz	370	24	58
Medallion of veal sauté (veal loin, mushrooms, cream sauce)	4 oz	535	35	59
Osso buco (braised veal)	1 shank	875	39	40
Roast veal	3 oz	145	5	31
Saltimbocca	2 rolls	415	21	45
Stir-fried veal w/ peppers	8 oz	385	29	68
Swiss-style shredded veal (w/ mushrooms, shallots, cream sauce)	6 oz	415	26	32
Veal chop in sour cream	1 chop	345	19	50
Veal Cordon Bleu (veal, ham, Swiss cheese)	4 oz	440	27	55
Veal curry	6 oz	390	26	60

	AMOUNT	CALORIES	FAT-GRAMS	% FAT
Veal cutlet:	4 oz	285	12	38
Breaded	4 oz	385	15	35
Italienne (cutlet, peppers, tomato sauce)	4 oz	325	14	39
Marsala (cutlet, prosciutto, mushrooms, wine sauce)	1 cutlet	455	31	62
Messina-style (sautéed veal, bread, ham, tomato sauce)	1 cutlet	530	28	48
Swiss-style (sautéed veal, tomatoes, mushrooms)	1 cutlet	360	11	28
Veal fricassee	8 oz	450	21	42
Veal goulash	6 oz	305	15	44
Veal kidneys in red wine	5 oz	265	19	64
Veal Marengo (veal, pasta, mushrooms, tomato sauce)	6 oz	340	12	31
Veal Marsala	4 oz	285	20	63
Veal meatballs (w/ tomato sauce & ½ cup rice)	8 oz	430	22	46
Veal Oscar (w/ crab, asparagus, Hollandaise sauce)	4 oz	910	73	72
Veal Parmigiana (cutlet, mozzarella, tomato sauce, Parmesan)	6 oz	590	30	46

	AMOUNT	CALORIES	FAT-GRAMS	% FAT
Veal piccata	4 oz	265	12	41
Veal Piemontese (sautéed veal, artichokes, cream sauce)	6 oz	480	39	73
Veal Provençal (sautéed veal, cream, Madeira sauce)	1 cutlet	280	16	51
Veal roll (w/ bacon & sour cream)	1 roll	460	36	71
Veal scallopini	8 oz	590	29	44
Veal scallops & rice casserole (w/ onions, celery, carrots & peas)	8 oz	285	10	32
Veal schnitzel (4-oz patties)	2 patties	425	30	64
Veal steak w/ eggplant (mozzarella & tomato sauce)	4 oz	755	63	75
Veal stew	8 oz	240	7	26
Veal sweetbread	2 pcs	765	25	29
Wiener schnitzel	4 oz	425	30	64

PASTA DISHES

(The pasta dishes in this section are based on cooked yields. A 5-ounce portion of cooked pasta measures approximately 1 cup; a 4-ounce portion of sauce measures approximately ½ cup. The combination of 5 ounces of pasta and 4 ounces of sauce, yielding a 9-ounce portion, is a modest serving. In many restaurants, the portion served might be one and a half to two times that size.)

	AMOUNT	CALORIES	FAT-GRAMS	% FAT
Cannelloni	10 oz	625	37	53
Kuchen, cheese	8 oz	440	21	43
Kugel w/ raisins	4 oz	395	12	27
Lasagna:				
Seafood lasagna (pasta, halibut, salmon, shrimp, vegetables, tomato sauce, 2 oz cheese)	10 oz	620	38	55
Traditional lasagna (pasta, meat sauce, ricotta, mozzarella)	10 oz	625	37	53

	AMOUNT	CALORIES	FAT-GRAMS	% FAT
Macaroni:				
Calico macaroni (pasta, tomato, bacon, peas, cheese) (4″ x 6″)	1 serving	270	9	30
Cheese & tomato casserole	6 oz	240	11	41
Macaroni & cheese	¾ cup	315	19	54
Macaroni-stuffed green pepper w/ cheese	1	335	19	51
Macaroni-stuffed tomato w/ cheese	1	340	19	50
Manicotti (pasta, cottage cheese, Parmesan, spinach, tomato sauce, mozzarella)	10 oz	720	24	30
Mostaccioli w/ gorgonzola & tomatoes	10 oz	540	19	32
Noodles:				
Buttered noodles	3 oz	135	3	20
Noodles Alfredo (w/ cream sauce)	9 oz	1,000	61	55
Noodles Lyonnaise (w/ butter & Parmesan)	3 oz	130	4	27
Noodles Mizar (w/ cottage cheese & sour cream)	3 oz	165	8	43
Noodles Romanoff (w/ sour cream, butter & Parmesan)	1 cup	325	22	61

	AMOUNT	CALORIES	FAT-GRAMS	% FAT
Noodle, salmon & mushroom casserole	12 oz	595	32	48
Poppy seed noodles (w/ butter & slivered almonds)	3 oz	160	6	34
Tuna noodle casserole	8 oz	300	12	36
Noodles, Oriental-style:				
Bahmi Goreng (meat, Chinese noodles, vegetables)	main dish	465	16	31
w/ peanut sauce	*add per 1 tbsp*	40	3	68
Bean threads, braised w/ pork & vegetables (Ants on a Tree)	main dish	395	21	48
Chop suey				
w/ chicken	8 oz	255	10	35
w/ pork	8 oz	195	10	46
Chow mein				
Beef	1 cup	300	17	51
Chicken	1 cup	255	10	35
Pork	6 oz	270	18	60
Seafood, meat & vegetable				
Pan-fried	main dish	680	36	48
w/ soft noodles	12 oz	565	30	48
Shrimp	1 cup	220	10	41
Chow mein noodles	½ cup	230	5	20
Oriental noodles, no fat added	1 cup	95	1	9

	AMOUNT	CALORIES	FAT-GRAMS	% FAT
Oriental noodles w/ chicken, shiitake mushrooms & sauce	10 oz	425	31	66
Oriental noodles w/ pork & peanut sauce	main dish	580	25	39
Pasta w/ chicken & vegetables in Szechuan sauce	12 oz	615	22	32
Rice noodles w/ pork, shrimp & vegetables	main dish	565	30	48
Szechuan noodles w/ Chinese cabbage & snow peas	8 oz	305	16	47
Szechuan noodles w/ Chinese cabbage, snow peas & scallops	10 oz	405	30	66
Thai noodles w/ pork, shrimp & chicken	main dish	555	15	24
Pansotti w/ butter sauce	10 oz	605	30	45
Pasta:				
Plain (5 oz)	1 cup	210	1	4
w/ anchovies, garlic & olive oil	9 oz	705	30	38
w/ beans	1 cup	300	8	24
w/ chicken & mushrooms in cream sauce	12 oz	1,145	64	50

	AMOUNT	CALORIES	FAT-GRAMS	% FAT
w/ chicken & pancetta in spicy red sauce topped w/ mozzarella	14 oz	975	55	51
w/ cream sauce & prosciutto	12 oz	1,040	61	53
w/ cream sauce & seafood (mussels, scallops, clams, crab)	12 oz	1,260	63	45
w/ cream sauce, salmon & sun-dried tomatoes	12 oz	1,200	79	59
w/ eggplant, tomatoes, garlic, cheese & olive oil	12 oz	705	30	38
w/ fresh tomatoes, basil & garlic	12 oz	520	11	19
w/ fresh tomatoes, basil, garlic & olive oil	12 oz	760	39	46
w/ ham, peas, Parmesan & butter	10 oz	555	21	34
w/ Italian sausage, spaghetti sauce & Sicilian peppers	14 oz	595	30	46
w/ marinara sauce	10 oz	295	5	15
w/ marinara & mushroom sauce	10 oz	410	14	31
w/ meatballs & tomato sauce (5 oz pasta, 5 oz sauce, 2 small meatballs)	13 oz	630	25	36

	AMOUNT	CALORIES	FAT-GRAMS	% FAT
w/ meat sauce (5 oz pasta, 5 oz sauce)	10 oz	410	14	31
w/ meat sauce, mozzarella & Parmesan	8 oz	405	22	49
w/ mushrooms & light cream sauce	1 cup	280	13	42
w/ pesto & seafood (clams, mussels, scallops, crab)	12 oz	1,010	45	42
w/ pesto sauce & Parmesan	9 oz	760	45	53
w/ prawns in garlic, wine & plum tomatoes	14 oz	915	42	41
w/ red clam sauce	14 oz	785	30	34
w/ spicy red sauce & seafood (mussels, clams, scallops, crab)	12 oz	545	7	11
w/ sweet peppers, basil, tomato & olive oil	¾ cup	170	8	42
w/ tomato sauce, meatless	10 oz	320	6	17
w/ tomatoes in spicy sauce (crushed red peppers) & Romano	¾ cup	290	9	25
w/ tomatoes in spicy sauce w/ pancetta	10 oz	655	39	54
w/ tuna, anchovies, olives, tomatoes, olive oil & mozzarella	12 oz	695	26	34

	AMOUNT	CALORIES	FAT-GRAMS	% FAT
w/ veal in cream sauce	14 oz	665	25	34
w/ white clam sauce	14 oz	985	47	43
Pasta all'Amatriciana (pasta, bacon, olive oil, white wine, tomatoes, Romano)	10 oz	655	39	53
Pasta alla Carbonara	9 oz	675	34	45
Pasta alla Francese (pasta, ham, peas, Parmesan, butter)	10 oz	555	21	34
Pasta alla Puttanesca (pasta, tomato sauce, olives, capers, garlic, basil)	8 oz	440	15	30
Pasta alla Romana (pasta, bacon, butter, Romano)	9 oz	675	34	45
Pasta Bolognese (5 oz pasta, 5 oz sauce)	10 oz	410	14	31
Pasta Capperei (pasta, tomato sauce, olives, capers, garlic, basil)	8 oz	440	15	30
Pasta e fagioli (pasta & beans)	1 cup	300	8	24
Pasta Florentine (pasta, spinach, pine nuts, anchovies, béchamel sauce)	14 oz	685	23	30

	AMOUNT	CALORIES	FAT-GRAMS	% FAT
Pasta primavera (pasta, broccoli, carrots, onion, peas, olive oil, Parmesan)	8 oz	425	20	42
in cream sauce	12 oz	1,200	75	56
w/ chicken	8 oz	475	20	38
w/ ham	8 oz	475	23	43
w/ salami (pasta, cauliflower, zucchini, sweet peppers, onion, tomato, olive oil, salami, Parmesan)	8 oz	520	35	60
Pasta quattroformaggi (w/ four cheeses: Gorgonzola, mozzarella, Gruyère, Parmesan)	1 cup	540	31	52
Pastitsio (pasta, ground lamb, tomato sauce, egg sauce, Parmesan)	10 oz	605	41	61
Penne all'Arrabiata (pasta, spicy tomato sauce, pancetta)	10 oz	490	15	28
Ravioli (10 spinach ravioli, 6 oz sauce)				
w/ Alfredo sauce	1 serving	1,165	51	40
w/ red sauce	1 serving	630	15	21
w/ tomato meat sauce	1 serving	740	23	28

	AMOUNT	CALORIES	FAT-GRAMS	% FAT
Shells:				
Baked shells (Fontina cheese, shrimp)	10 oz	450	21	42
Seafood-stuffed shells (cottage cheese, milk, celery, zucchini, onion, shrimp, crab)	3 shells	300	6	18
Shells w/ white clam sauce	9 oz	455	6	12
Spaetzle	4 oz	275	10	32
Tortellini:				
& vegetable confetti	9 oz	435	23	48
w Alfredo sauce (10 spinach tortellini, 6 oz sauce)	1 serving	1,165	51	40
w/ red sauce (10 spinach tortellini, 6 oz sauce)	1 serving	630	15	21
w/ tomato/meat sauce (10 spinach tortellini, 6 oz sauce)	1 serving	740	23	28
Vermicelli Ballerini (pasta, olive oil, walnuts, powdered sugar, nutmeg, allspice)	6 oz	880	26	26

PIZZA

	AMOUNT	CALORIES	FAT-GRAMS	% FAT
Calzone:				
Mushroom & prosciutto	1	540	25	42
Sausage & mushroom	1	520	25	43
Pizza:				
Pesto pizza	1 slice of 7" pie	500	32	57
Pizza alla Napoletana (tomato-cheese pizza)	1 slice of 7" pie	305	14	41
White pizza	1/5 of 12" pie	365	16	39
Pizza add-ons:				
Artichoke hearts	1 oz	30	2	60
Black olives	1 oz	30	3	90
Canadian bacon	1 oz	45	2	40
Green peppers	1 oz	5	0	0
Ground beef	1 oz	80	6	67
Italian sausage	1 oz	90	8	80
Jalapeño peppers	1 oz	10	0	0
Mushrooms	1 oz	10	0	0
Onions	1 oz	10	0	0
Pepperoni	1 oz	140	13	84
Pineapple tidbits	½ cup	50	0	0
Salami	1 oz	110	10	82

POULTRY & POULTRY DISHES

CHICKEN	AMOUNT	CALORIES	FAT-GRAMS	% FAT
Arroz con pollo	1 serving	515	25	43
Baked chicken:	1 quarter	340	22	58
Greek-style (w/ potatoes, onions, lemon sauce)	1 quarter	575	30	47
w/ orzo (1 cup)	1 quarter	645	35	49
Batter-fried chicken	1 quarter	455	27	53
BBQ chicken	1 quarter	405	25	56
Blackened chicken	½ breast	285	17	54
Black mushroom chicken	main dish	295	15	46
Boiled chicken	1 quarter	240	9	34
Broiled chicken	1 half	665	41	55
Spicy hot	1 quarter	365	22	54
Brunswick stew	10 oz	315	13	37
Cajun chicken	4 oz	285	17	54
Chicken à la king	6 oz	225	13	51
Chicken & chips (2.7 oz chicken, 3 oz fries)	1 serving	400	22	51

	AMOUNT	CALORIES	FAT-GRAMS	% FAT
Chicken & dumpling (1 pc chicken, 1 dumpling, sauce)	main dish	375	23	55
Chicken & peppers (½ breast w/ peppers)	1 serving	225	10	40
Chicken & rice casserole	8 oz	280	7	22
Chicken breast fillet				
w/ skin	½ breast	195	8	37
w/o skin	½ breast	140	3	21
Chicken breast w/ prosciutto & fontina	½ breast	245	12	44
Chicken burgoo	10 oz	495	16	29
Chicken Cacciatori	10 oz	250	13	46
Chicken Calvados	½ breast	305	19	56
Chicken Cordon Bleu	1 breast	800	50	56
Chicken Creole	8 oz	275	11	36
Chicken crepes w/ cream sauce	2	875	51	52
Chicken croquettes (2 oz each)	2	350	16	41
Chicken curry	6 oz	255	15	52
Chicken Diavola (breaded chicken breast, Parmesan, Dijon sauce)	main dish	625	28	40
Chicken Dijon (w/ 2 oz Dijon cream sauce)	½ breast	405	17	37
Chicken Divan	6 oz	385	18	42
Chicken fricassee	6 oz	260	16	56
Chicken-fried steak	3 oz	370	27	66

	AMOUNT	CALORIES	FAT-GRAMS	% FAT
Chicken Jack Daniel's	½ breast	300	19	56
Chicken Jambalaya	8 oz	340	12	32
Chicken kabobs	1 kabob	273	10	33
Chicken Kiev	1 breast	730	42	52
Chicken liver sauté	6 oz	255	14	49
Chicken livers hunter-style (w/ tomatoes, tomato paste, mushrooms, onions)	6 oz	260	14	48
Chicken loaf w/ fricassee sauce	6 oz	380	20	47
Chicken Lorraine (w/ mushrooms, artichokes, cream sauce)	1 breast	775	50	58
Chicken Marsala	4 oz	445	26	52
Chicken Nogada (chicken breast, almonds, mushrooms, sauce)	4 oz	530	40	68
Chicken nuggets	½ breast	505	22	39
Chicken Oscar	4 oz	870	67	69
Chicken paprika w/ noodles (1 quarter chicken, 3 oz noodles/ sauce)	1 serving	595	28	42
Chicken paprikash (chicken, sour cream sauce)	1 quarter	455	30	59
Chicken Parmigiana	1 breast	625	28	40
Chicken pasta primavera	1½ cups	290	12	37

POULTRY/POULTRY DISHES

	AMOUNT	CALORIES	FAT-GRAMS	% FAT
Chicken patties ½ breast w/o skin):				
Fried	1 serving	290	19	59
Grilled	1 serving	140	3	19
Chicken piccata	4 oz	415	25	54
Chicken pilaf (1 quarter chicken, 8 oz pilaf)	1 serving	715	44	55
Chicken Polynesian (w/ vegetables, sweet & sour sauce)	8 oz	285	17	54
Chicken Portugal (marinated in olive oil, grilled)	4 oz	290	19	59
Chicken pot pie	8 oz	800	60	67
Chicken Royal Hawaiian (w/ mushrooms, almonds, coconut)	6 oz	400	27	60
Chicken saltimbocca	1 breast	800	50	56
Chicken soufflé	5½ oz	295	19	58
Chicken stew	10 oz	315	13	37
Chicken-stuffed baked tomato	2 halves	255	12	42
Chicken tetrazzini	8 oz	460	18	35
Chicken w/ black bean sauce	6 oz	320	18	51
Chicken w/ olives & pine nuts	3 oz	285	18	57
Coq au vin	1 quarter	505	35	62
Coq au vin sauté	½ breast	315	11	31
Crab-filled breast of chicken w/ Hollandaise sauce	1 pc	735	67	82

	AMOUNT	CALORIES	FAT-GRAMS	% FAT
Creamed chicken	6 oz	275	16	52
& ham on corn bread	8 oz	560	27	44
& vegetables on				
biscuit	6 oz	445	24	48
Escalloped chicken				
& noodles	8 oz	315	14	40
Fried chicken	2 pcs	525	28	48
Garlic chicken	main dish	365	10	25
Ginger chicken	main dish	375	10	24
Green pepper chicken	main dish	295	15	46
Lemon chicken				
(3 oz grilled breast,				
2 oz lemon sauce)	1 serving	290	14	43
Malibu chicken				
(1 breast, ham,				
cheese, mustard				
sauce	main dish	800	50	56
Mesquite grilled				
chicken (½ breast				
w/o skin, basted				
w/ olive oil)	1 serving	215	5	22
Mexican-style chicken:				
Chimichanga				
(chicken, cheese,				
tortilla, sour cream)	1	605	35	52
Enchilada (enchilada,				
sour cream sauce)	1	575	33	52
Enchilada verde				
& sour cream	1	450	30	60
Fajita (chicken, peppers,				
onion, tortilla)	1	415	21	45
w/ cheese,				
guacamole				
& sour cream	1	780	44	51

	AMOUNT	CALORIES	FAT-GRAMS	% FAT
Flauta (tortilla, chicken filling)	1	225	10	40
Quesadilla	1	375	17	41
Sopito (chicken, lettuce, tomato, cheese)	1	435	21	44
Taco (w/ cheese, avocado & salsa)	1	435	21	44
Tostada (chicken, beans, cheese, olives, avocado, sour cream)	1	935	55	52
Paella	1 quarter	675	28	37
Pine nut chicken (w/ brandy cream sauce)	4 oz	530	40	68
Roast chicken w/ new potatoes	1 quarter	550	28	46
Roast chicken w/ rosemary	4 oz	285	10	34
Rotisserie chicken	1 half	665	41	55
Smothered chicken (w/ onion, mushrooms, cream sauce)	½ breast	775	50	58
Snow White chicken	main dish	295	15	46
Stuffed chicken breast (bread stuffing, sauce)	1 breast	395	26	59
Oriental-style chicken:				
Almond chicken	main dish	580	38	59
Cashew chicken	main dish	580	36	57
Chicken & snow peas	main dish	295	15	46

	AMOUNT	CALORIES	FAT-GRAMS	% FAT
Chicken chop suey	8 oz	185	8	38
Chicken chow mein	6 oz	180	8	40
Chicken teriyaki	1 quarter	355	17	43
Hot & sour chicken	main dish	300	15	45
Kung Pao chicken	8 oz	490	25	46
Stir-fried chicken				
w/ eggplant	main dish	385	20	46
w/ vegetables	6 oz	245	14	51
Sweet & sour chicken	8 oz	305	6	18
Thai-style chicken	main dish	320	17	48

CORNISH GAME HEN

	AMOUNT	CALORIES	FAT-GRAMS	% FAT
Baked Cornish game hen	½ hen	400	25	56
Orange-glazed Cornish game hen w/ wild rice stuffing	1 bird	560	26	42

DUCK

	AMOUNT	CALORIES	FAT-GRAMS	% FAT
Roast duck	1 quarter	835	69	75
À l'orange	1 half	1,745	139	72
Szechuan duck (½ duck)	13.4 oz	1,285	108	75

GOOSE

	AMOUNT	CALORIES	FAT-GRAMS	% FAT
Roast goose	6 oz	360	25	63
Roast goose Provençal	9 oz	730	48	59

	AMOUNT	CALORIES	FAT-GRAMS	% FAT

PHEASANT

	AMOUNT	CALORIES	FAT-GRAMS	% FAT
Roast pheasant w/ sausage dressing	1 quarter	1,105	69	56
Roast pheasant w/ wild rice dressing (8 oz pheasant, ½ cup dressing)	1 serving	860	44	46

QUAIL

	AMOUNT	CALORIES	FAT-GRAMS	% FAT
Roast quail (4 oz quail)	2 birds	500	36	65

TURKEY

	AMOUNT	CALORIES	FAT-GRAMS	% FAT
Baked turkey legs	1 leg	420	13	30
Cranberry-sauced turkey steaks	4 oz	255	8	28
Grilled turkey piccata	6 oz	265	9	31
Roast turkey	6 oz	385	18	42
Turkey & biscuit	6 oz	395	20	46
Turkey Divan	8 oz	630	33	47
Turkey meatballs (1″ each)	3	325	14	38
Turkey mole	10 oz	530	26	44
Turkey wings Creole	1 wing	450	25	50

RICE & OTHER GRAINS

(For rice dishes made with beans, see VEGETABLES. The rice dishes in this section are based on cooked yields. A 3-ounce portion of cooked rice measures approximately ½ cup.)

	AMOUNT	CALORIES	FAT-GRAMS	% FAT
Barley w/ mushrooms	3 oz	180	5	25
Bulgur w/ Parmesan	⅔ cup	190	3	13
Chop suey:				
w/ chicken	8 oz	255	10	35
w/ pork	8 oz	195	10	46
Corn fritters				
(1.5 oz each)	2	120	3	23
Cornmeal:				
Fried polenta				
(2 oz each)	2 slices	295	16	49
Hush puppies				
(1.5 oz each)	2	140	5	32
Couscous (no fat added)	⅔ cup	110	1	7
Dressings/stuffings:				
Bread (½ cup)	3 oz	290	12	37
Chestnut	3 oz	225	11	44
Corn bread	3 oz	240	12	45
& sausage	4 oz	250	17	61
Oyster corn bread	3 oz	185	11	53

	AMOUNT	CALORIES	FAT-GRAMS	% FAT
Sausage	3 oz	260	9	31
Wild rice	4 oz	230	9	35
Dumpling (1.5 oz)	1	115	3	23
Grits:				
No fat added	1 cup	145	0	0
w/ 2 tsp butter	1 cup	225	8	72
Grits au gratin	½ cup	190	12	56
Matzo cakes				
(w/ olive oil)	4 oz	250	20	72
Polenta:				
Baked polenta				
(w/ fontina,				
Gorgonzola)	1 slice	625	32	46
Soft polenta				
w/ bacon				
& rosemary	1 serving	185	8	38
w/ sausage	1 serving	360	16	40
Rice:				
Baked rice	side dish	330	13	35
Browned rice	3 oz	160	5	28
Cajun dirty rice	1½ cup	315	19	54
Cheese rice				
croquettes				
(3 oz each)	2	520	23	40
Curried rice	3 oz	150	6	36
Fried rice	3 oz	140	4	26
Herbed rice				
(no fat added)	3 oz	110	1	8
Maui rice	8 oz	395	15	34
Rice & bean sprouts	1 cup	295	7	21
Rice & mushrooms	3 oz	130	5	34
Rice Calcutta	3 oz	105	3	25
Rice, peas &				
pancetta	5 oz	380	10	24

	AMOUNT	CALORIES	FAT-GRAMS	% FAT
Rice pilaf	3 oz	150	6	36
Greek-style	6 oz	330	10	27
Turkish-style (w/ pine nuts & almonds)	6 oz	420	20	43
Rice pilaf & spinach	12 oz	310	11	32
Tomato fried rice	4 oz	170	9	48
Risotto:	4 oz	215	7	29
Risotto primavera	10 oz	460	20	39
Wild mushroom risotto	6 oz	395	15	34
Saffron rice	3 oz	150	6	30
Spanish rice	4 oz	115	3	23
White rice (w/ ½ tsp butter)	3 oz	115	2	15
Wild rice casserole	3 oz	125	5	36

SALADS & DRESSINGS

SALADS	AMOUNT	CALORIES	FAT-GRAMS	% FAT
(Dressing included unless otherwise noted.)				
Ambrosia fruit salad	side dish	215	2	8
Antipasto platter	side dish	230	15	59
Apple & date salad	1 cup	310	19	55
Apple & grape salad	1 cup	265	19	64
Apple-grape aspic w/ walnuts	5 oz	140	4	25
Apricot, banana & grape salad (no dressing)	1 cup	85	0	0
Apricot parfait salad	1 serving	185	9	44
Artichoke, avocado & orange salad	1 artichoke	300	20	60
Asparagus vinaigrette	3 spears	60	6	77
Asparagus & egg	side dish	205	16	70
Asparagus & tomato salad	side dish	125	10	73
Avocado, tomato & chicken salad (no dressing)	1 cup	175	9	47
Banana-berry salad	side dish	110	0	0

	AMOUNT	CALORIES	FAT-GRAMS	% FAT
Beef salads:				
Beef & apple salad	main dish	345	19	49
Beef & broccoli salad	main dish	310	21	61
Beef & fruit salad	main dish	400	24	54
Beef & vegetable stir-fry salad	main dish	240	12	45
Beef, pasta & bean salad	main dish	365	13	32
Beef salad w/ vegetables	1.5 cup	255	14	49
Marinated steak salad w/ shiitake mushrooms	main dish	325	23	63
Pasta, beef & vegetable salad	main dish	525	34	58
Steak salad	main dish	330	21	57
Taco salad	1.5 cup	455	37	73
Belgian endive salad	1 head	205	21	92
Broccoli & egg salad	side dish	340	30	80
Broccoli & tomato salad	side dish	265	24	82
Cabbage, carrots & green pepper salad (no dressing)	1 cup	35	0	0
Caesar salad	main dish	415	40	86
Cardinal salad (3" x 3")	1 serving	100	0	0
Carrot & raisin salad	1 cup	375	28	67
Carrot, apple & raisin salad	1 cup	390	28	64
Carrot, pineapple & raisin salad	1 cup	405	29	71
Cauliflower & tomato salad	side dish	270	23	77

	AMOUNT	CALORIES	FAT GRAMS	% FAT
Chef's salad bowl (no dressing)	1.5 cup	365	32	79
Cherry crunch salad (3" x 3")	1 serving	185	2	10
Chicken salads:				
Chicken almond salad	1 cup	385	32	75
Chicken & pasta salad	main dish	455	23	45
Chicken artichoke salad	main dish	410	26	57
Chicken, avocado & tomato (no dressing)	1.5 cup	175	9	47
Chicken bulgur salad (no dressing)	main dish	250	4	14
Chicken Caesar salad	main dish	550	48	78
Chicken fajita salad	main dish	365	14	34
w/ 1 tbsp guacamole	add	50	6	100
w/ 1 tbsp sour cream	add	25	3	100
w/ 1 tbsp tomato salsa	add	5	0	0
Chicken-filled melon (no dressing)	main dish	250	4	14
Chicken salad "Fat Watcher"	main dish	240	5	19
Chicken salad w/ tortellini & sun-dried tomatoes	main dish	510	20	35

	AMOUNT	CALORIES	FAT-GRAMS	% FAT
Chicken salad				
w/ wild rice	main dish	430	19	40
Chicken spinach				
salad	main dish	370	27	65
w/ chutney	main dish	460	28	55
Chicken taco salad	main dish	425	26	55
Curried chicken				
cashew salad	main dish	625	45	65
Fried chicken &				
spinach salad	main dish	370	27	65
Grilled chicken &				
vegetable salad				
(no dressing)	main dish	245	9	33
Grilled chicken				
Waldorf salad	main dish	460	28	55
Hot chicken salad				
w/ honey mustard				
dressing	main dish	505	34	60
Peking chicken salad				
(no dressing)	main dish	230	7	27
Sesame chicken				
& rice salad	main dish	330	15	41
Stir-fry chicken				
salad	main dish	410	34	74
Thai chicken salad				
(no dressing)	main dish	310	6	18
Tomato stuffed				
w/ chicken salad	1	265	17	58
Chinese cabbage salad	1 cup	110	6	49
Cobb salad	main dish	495	36	65
Coleslaw	1 cup	210	13	56
Cottage cheese				
& chives	½ cup	115	5	39
Cottage cheese & fruit	1 serving	195	5	23

	AMOUNT	CALORIES	FAT-GRAMS	% FAT
Cottage cheese & vegetables	¼ cup	45	2	38
Couscous salad	side dish	275	15	49
Crab Louie	main dish	590	47	71
Crab salad w/ melon	main dish	360	23	57
Cucumber & onion salad	1 cup	165	14	76
Cucumber-lime salad, molded (3″ x 3″)	1 serving	80	2	22
Cucumbers in sour cream	1 cup	135	9	60
Curried chicken cashew salad	main dish	625	45	65
Duck salad	main dish	450	32	64
w/ fruit		640	41	58
Fajita salad	main dish	365	14	34
w/ 1 tbsp guacamole	add	50	6	100
w/ 1 tbsp sour cream	add	25	3	100
w/ 1 tbsp tomato salsa	add	5	0	0
Fried chicken & spinach salad	main dish	370	27	65
Fruit salads:				
Ambrosia fruit salad	side dish	215	2	8
Apple & date salad	1 cup	310	19	55
Apple & grape salad	1 cup	265	19	64
Apple-grape aspic w/ walnuts	5 oz	140	4	25
Apricot, banana & grape salad (no dressing)	1 cup	85	0	0
Apricot parfait salad	1 serving	185	9	44

	AMOUNT	CALORIES	FAT-GRAMS	% FAT
Artichoke, avocado & orange salad	1 artichoke	300	20	60
Avocado, orange & grapefruit salad	side dish	340	31	82
Banana-berry salad	side dish	110	0	0
Beef & apple salad	main dish	345	19	49
Beef & fruit salad	main dish	400	24	54
Carrot & raisin salad	1 cup	375	28	67
Carrot, apple & raisin salad	1 cup	390	28	64
Carrot, pineapple & raisin salad	1 cup	405	29	71
Cherry crunch salad (3" x 3")	1 serving	185	2	10
Chicken-filled melons (no dressing)	main dish	250	4	14
Cottage cheese & fruit	1 serving	195	5	23
Couscous salad	side dish	275	15	49
Cucumber-lime salad (3" x 3")	1 serving	80	2	22
Crab salad w/ melon	main dish	360	23	57
Duck salad w/ fruit	main dish	640	41	58
Fruit & cream cheese	½ cup	170	4	21
Fruit marshmallow	½ cup	120	4	30
Fruit plate (fruit only)	side dish	230	0	0
Fruit platter w/ 1 oz cheese wedge	1 serving	320	10	28
Fruit salad				
w/ avocado	1 serving	300	16	48
w/ cottage cheese	1 serving	195	5	23
w/ creamy dressing	1 cup	245	18	67

	AMOUNT	CALORIES	FAT-GRAMS	% FAT
Grapefruit basket	1 serving	190	0	0
Grapefruit salad	½ cup	76	0	0
Grilled chicken				
Waldorf salad	main dish	460	28	55
Hazelnut, pear &				
arugula salad	side dish	110	9	73
Jellied cranberry				
& apple	½ cup	205	0	0
Jellied cranberry				
relish	½ cup	205	0	0
Jellied fruit	½ cup	100	0	0
Lime-pear aspic				
(3" x 3")	1 serving	95	0	0
Lobster-melon salad	main dish	375	20	48
Melon salad	1 cup	55	0	0
Molded fruit salads.				
See Molded salads.				
Peach half stuffed				
w/ cream cheese	1 serving	95	3	29
Pineapple boat fruit				
salad	1 serving	255	0	0
Pineapple-lime salad	½ cup	145	7	43
Pineapple ring				
& stuffed dates	1 serving	60	3	44
Regal fruit salad w/				
whipped topping	½ cup	150	7	41
Ribbon mold	½ cup	290	16	50
Scallop salad				
w/ fruit salsa				
(no dressing)	side dish	120	1	7
Spinach chutney				
salad	main dish	460	28	55
Summer fruit salad	1 cup	90	0	0
Tropical fruit salad	1 cup	100	0	0

	AMOUNT	CALORIES	FAT-GRAMS	% FAT
Tropical fruits w/ lime syrup	1 cup	120	0	0
Waldorf salad	1 cup	255	15	52
Waldorf salad mold	½ cup	135	4	26
Winter fruit salad	1 cup	115	0	0
Gado-gado	side dish	280	21	68
Garden primavera salad (no dressing)	1 cup	15	0	0
Grapefruit basket	1 serving	190	0	0
Grapefruit salad	½ cup	76	0	0
Greek salad	side dish	180	15	75
Greek-style pasta salad	main dish	405	30	66
Green salad:	1 cup	150	15	89
w/ fresh basil, mozzarella, tomato (no dressing)	side dish	270	15	50
w/ chèvre (goat cheese)	side dish	345	26	68
Grilled chicken & vegetable salad (no dressing)	main dish	245	9	33
Grilled chicken Waldorf salad	main dish	460	28	55
Grilled swordfish salad (w/ olives, onion, oranges, arugula)	main dish	450	31	65
Ham & cheese platter w/ potato salad	side dish	390	24	56
Ham & rice salad	1 cup	370	10	24
Ham salad platter w/ potato chips	1 serving	595	45	68
Hearts of palm salad	side dish	95	7	66

	AMOUNT	CALORIES	FAT-GRAMS	% FAT
Hot chicken salad w/ honey mustard dressing	main dish	505	34	60
Hot curried pork salad	main dish	410	25	55
Jellied cranberry & apple	½ cup	205	0	0
Jellied cranberry relish	½ cup	205	0	0
Jellied fruit	½ cup	100	0	0
Lamb brochette salad	main dish	465	26	50
Layered 24-hour salad	side dish	365	35	86
Lime-pear aspic (3" x 3")	1 serving	95	0	0
Lobster-melon salad	main dish	375	20	48
Macaroni & ham salad	1 cup	390	22	51
Macaroni salad	1 cup	360	18	45
Marinated broccoli	side dish	110	10	82
Marinated cauliflower	½ cup	110	10	83
Marinated cucumber salad	½ cup	115	9	70
Marinated garden salad	1 cup	230	17	74
Marinated green bean salad	side dish	205	20	88
Marinated mixed vegetable salad	1 cup	230	17	74
Marinated mushroom salad	side dish	90	7	71
Marinated steak salad w/ shiitake mushrooms	main dish	330	23	63
Marinated vegetable & cheese salad	side dish	255	24	85
Melon salad	1 cup	55	0	0

	AMOUNT	CALORIES	FAT-GRAMS	% FAT
Molded salads:				
Apple-grape aspic w/ walnuts	5 oz	140	4	25
Apricot parfait salad	1 serving	185	9	44
Cardinal salad (3" x 3")	1 serving	100	0	0
Cherry crunch salad (3" x 3")	1 serving	185	2	10
Cucumber-lime salad (3" x 3")	1 serving	80	2	22
Fruit & cream cheese	½ cup	170	4	21
Fruit marshmallow	½ cup	120	4	30
Jellied cranberry & apple	½ cup	205	0	0
Jellied cranberry relish	½ cup	205	0	0
Jellied fruit	½ cup	100	0	0
Lime-pear aspic (3" x 3")	1 serving	95	0	0
Molded Bing cherry salad w/ walnuts	½ cup	145	4	25
Molded citrus salad	1 serving	95	0	0
Molded creamy lime salad	½ cup	160	6	34
Molded mandarin orange salad	5 oz	95	0	0
Perfection salad	½ cup	105	0	0
Pineapple-lime salad	½ cup	145	7	43
Regal fruit salad w/ whipped topping	½ cup	150	7	41
Ribbon mold	½ cup	290	16	50
Seafood aspic	½ cup	70	1	13
Tomato aspic	½ cup	35	0	0

	AMOUNT	CALORIES	FAT-GRAMS	% FAT
Tuna mousse	½ cup	280	19	61
Waldorf salad mold	½ cup	135	4	26
Oriental noodle salad	main dish	300	8	24
Oriental salad	side dish	210	15	65
Pasta salads:				
Beef, pasta & bean salad	main dish	365	13	32
Chicken & pasta salad	main dish	455	23	45
Chicken salad w/ tortellini & sun-dried tomatoes	main dish	510	20	35
Greek-style pasta salad	main dish	405	30	66
Macaroni & ham salad	1 cup	390	22	51
Macaroni salad	1 cup	360	18	45
Oriental noodle salad	main dish	300	8	24
Pasta & bean salad	side dish	270	16	53
Pasta & salami salad	main dish	670	52	70
Pasta & shrimp salad	main dish	480	24	45
Pasta, beef & vegetable salad	main dish	530	34	58
Pasta, ham & cheese salad	main dish	490	25	46
Pasta primavera salad	1 cup	365	27	67
Pasta salad	1 cup	360	18	45
Peking chicken salad (no dressing)	main dish	230	7	27
Pesto pasta salad	1 cup	400	26	58
Salmon & pasta salad	main dish	485	31	57

	AMOUNT	CALORIES	FAT-GRAMS	% FAT
Seafood pasta salad	main dish	480	24	45
Tortellini salad	main dish	580	40	62
Tortellini shrimp salad	main dish	560	32	51
Trio salad platter	main dish	675	46	61
Turkey & vegetable salad	main dish	420	22	47
Turkey, black bean & pasta salad	main dish	570	30	47
Peach half stuffed w/ cream cheese	1 serving	93	3	29
Peking chicken salad (no dressing)	main dish	230	7	27
Perfection salad	½ cup	105	0	0
Pesto pasta salad	1 cup	400	26	58
Pickled beets	½ cup	95	0	0
w/ egg slices		135	3	20
w/ onions		105	0	0
Pineapple fruit boat salad	1 serving	255	0	0
Pineapple-lime salad	½ cup	145	7	43
Pineapple ring & stuffed dates	1 serving	60	3	44
Poached salmon & marinated vegetable platter	main dish	470	33	63
Pork salads:				
Chef's salad bowl (no dressing)	1.5 cup	365	32	79
Ham & cheese platter	1 serving	390	24	56
Ham & rice salad	1 cup	370	10	24
Ham salad platter w/ potato chips	1 serving	595	45	68

	AMOUNT	CALORIES	FAT-GRAMS	% FAT
Hot curried pork salad	main dish	410	25	55
Macaroni & ham salad	1 cup	390	22	51
Pasta, ham & cheese salad	main dish	490	25	46
Pork & cabbage salad	main dish	545	26	43
Pork & roasted pepper salad	main dish	310	23	66
Potato salads:				
Hot German potato salad	1 cup	250	16	58
Old-fashioned potato salad	1 cup	300	18	54
Potato salad w/ sliced Polish sausage (½ cup salad, 3 oz sausage)	1 serving	395	26	59
Salami-potato salad plate	main dish	640	43	60
Salmon & potato salad	main dish	615	40	59
Seafood & potato salad	main dish	485	29	54
Regal fruit salad w/ whipped topping	½ cup	150	7	41
Relish plate	1 serving	50	1	17
Ribbon mold	½ cup	290	16	50
Rice & avocado salad	side dish	285	20	64
Rice & vegetable salad	1 cup	305	17	50
Roasted pepper salad	side dish	75	5	58
Roasted pepper, tomato & olive salad	side dish	295	25	76

	AMOUNT	CALORIES	FAT-GRAMS	% FAT
Salami & pasta salad	main dish	670	52	70
Salami-potato salad plate	main dish	640	43	60
Salmon salads:				
Poached salmon & marinated vegetable platter	main dish	470	33	63
Salmon & pasta salad	main dish	485	31	57
Salmon & potato salad	main dish	615	40	59
Salmon salad	side dish	235	11	42
Smoked salmon platter	1 serving	240	9	34
Scallop salad w/ fruit salsa (no dressing)	side dish	120	1	7
Seafood salads:				
Crab Louie	main dish	590	47	71
Crab salad w/ melon	main dish	360	23	57
Grilled swordfish salad (w/ olives, onion, oranges, arugula)	main dish	450	31	65
Lobster-melon salad	main dish	375	20	48
Pasta & shrimp salad	main dish	480	24	45
Scallop salad w/ fruit salsa (no dressing)	main dish	120	1	7
Seafood & potato salad	main dish	485	29	54
Seafood aspic	½ cup	70	1	13
Seafood pasta salad	main dish	480	24	45
Seafood salad	main dish	650	49	68
Seviche salad	main dish	200	11	50

	AMOUNT	CALORIES	FAT-GRAMS	% FAT
Shrimp bowl (no dressing)	side dish	120	3	22
Shrimp Caesar salad	main dish	535	42	70
Shrimp Louie	1 serving	590	47	71
Shrimp salad Oriental-style	main dish	260	15	52
Shrimp salad sushi-style (no dressing)	main dish	195	2	10
Shrimp taco salad	main dish	650	49	68
Sole salad w/ asparagus & mixed greens	side dish	300	19	57
Tomato stuffed w/ tuna salad	1	175	11	56
Tortellini shrimp salad	main dish	560	32	51
Trio salad platter	main dish	675	46	61
Tuna fish & mixed vegetable salad	1 serving	425	32	67
Tuna fish chef's salad bowl (no dressing)	1.5 cup	345	31	81
Tuna-havarti salad	main dish	380	26	61
Tuna mousse	½ cup	280	19	61
Warm tuna salad	main dish	250	10	36
Wild rice & shrimp salad	main dish	260	15	52
Sesame chicken & rice salad	main dish	330	15	41
Seviche salad	main dish	200	11	50
Shrimp salads: Pasta & shrimp salad	main dish	480	24	45
Shrimp bowl (no dressing)	side dish	120	3	22

	AMOUNT	CALORIES	FAT-GRAMS	% FAT
Shrimp Caesar salad	main dish	535	42	70
Shrimp Louie	1 serving	590	47	71
Shrimp salad Oriental-style	main dish	260	15	52
Shrimp salad sushi-style (no dressing)	main dish	195	2	10
Shrimp taco salad	main dish	650	49	68
Tortellini shrimp salad	main dish	560	32	51
Wild rice & shrimp salad	main dish	260	15	52
Sole salad w/ asparagus & mixed greens	side dish	300	19	57
Spinach-chutney salad	main dish	460	28	55
Spinach salad (no dressing)	1 cup	255	6	21
w/ chicken (no dressing)	main dish	370	27	65
Steak salad	main dish	330	21	57
Stir-fry chicken salad	main dish	410	34	74
Stuffed head of lettuce	side dish	110	10	92
Summer fruit salad	1 cup	90	0	0
Tabbouleh salad	side dish	245	14	51
Taco salad	1.5 cup	455	37	73
w/ tostada shell		50	2	36
per ½ fresh avocado	*add*	155	14	82
per 1 tbsp guacamole	*add*	50	6	100
per 1 tbsp salsa	*add*	5	0	0
per 1 tbsp sour cream	*add*	25	3	100
Thai chicken salad (no dressing)	main dish	310	6	18
Three-bean salad	1 cup	310	14	41

	AMOUNT	CALORIES	FAT-GRAMS	% FAT
Tomato salads:				
Asparagus & tomato salad	side dish	125	10	73
Avocado, tomato & chicken salad (no dressing)	main dish	175	9	47
Broccoli & tomato salad	side dish	265	24	82
Cauliflower & tomato salad	side dish	270	23	77
Chicken, avocado & tomato (no dressing)	1.5 cup	175	9	47
Chicken salad w/ tortellini & sun-dried tomatoes	main dish	510	20	35
Green salad w/ fresh basil, mozzarella & tomato	side dish	270	15	50
Tomato à l'Andalouse	1 tomato	230	22	86
Tomato & avocado (no dressing)	side dish	90	8	78
Tomato & cucumber (no dressing)	side dish	25	0	0
Tomato & green pepper rings (no dressing)	side dish	20	0	0
Tomato & onion salad	1 cup	160	13	72
Tomato aspic	½ cup	35	0	0
Tomato salad	½ cup	80	6	67
Tomato stuffed w/ chicken salad	1	265	17	58

	AMOUNT	CALORIES	FAT-GRAMS	% FAT
Tomato stuffed w/ tuna salad	1	175	11	56
Tortellini salad	side dish	290	20	62
Tortellini shrimp salad	main dish	560	32	51
Tossed green salad (no dressing)	1 cup	15	0	0
Tossed greens w/ nasturtiums	side dish	115	11	85
Trio salad platter	main dish	675	46	61
Tropical fruit salad	1 cup	100	0	0
Tropical fruits w/ lime syrup	1 cup	120	0	0
Tuna fish & mixed vegetable salad	1 serving	425	32	67
Tuna fish chef's salad bowl (no dressing)	1.5 cup	345	31	81
Tuna-havarti salad	main dish	380	26	61
Tuna mousse	½ cup	280	19	61
Turkey & vegetable salad	main dish	420	22	47
Turkey, black bean & pasta salad	main dish	570	30	47
Turkey cold platter (no dressing)	main dish	375	6	19
Vegetable salad (no dressing)	1 cup	15	0	0
Vegetable salad à la Russe	1 cup	290	22	68
Vegetable tray	2 oz	40	0	0
Waldorf salad	1 cup	255	15	52
Waldorf salad mold	½ cup	135	4	26
Warm tuna salad	main dish	250	10	36
Wild rice & shrimp salad	main dish	260	15	52

	AMOUNT	CALORIES	FAT-GRAMS	% FAT
Wilted greens salad w/ bacon dressing	1 cup	255	28	99
Winter fruit salad (no dressing)	1 cup	115	0	0

SALAD BAR ADD-ONS

	AMOUNT	CALORIES	FAT-GRAMS	% FAT
Alfalfa sprouts	1 oz	10	0	0
American cheese	1 oz	105	9	75
Applesauce	1 cup	100	0	0
Bacon bits	½ oz	40	2	45
Banana chips	1 oz	100	0	0
Beets	1 cup	60	0	0
Blue cheese dressing	1 tbsp	80	8	90
Blueberries	1 tbsp	5	0	0
Bread sticks	2	35	1	28
Broccoli	½ cup	15	0	0
Cabbage	1 cup	15	0	0
Cantaloupe	2 pcs	15	0	0
Carrots	¼ cup	10	0	0
Cauliflower	½ cup	15	0	0
Cheddar cheese	1 oz	115	9	71
Cherry peppers	1 tbsp	5	0	0
Chow mein noodles	1 oz	140	6	38
Coconut	1 oz	160	11	62
Coleslaw	3.5 oz	70	4	51
Cottage cheese	½ cup	125	5	36
Crackers (saltines)	2	25	1	36
Croutons	½ oz	70	3	38
Cucumbers	4 slices	5	0	0
Eggs	1 egg	80	5	56
French-style dressing	1 tbsp	90	10	99
Garbanzo beans	½ cup	360	5	12

	AMOUNT	CALORIES	FAT-GRAMS	% FAT
Gelatine:				
Lime	½ cup	90	0	0
Strawberry	½ cup	90	0	0
Grapefruit sections	1 cup	80	0	0
Grapes	1 cup	100	0	0
Green peppers	¼ cup	10	0	0
Honeydew melon	2 pcs	25	0	0
Italian dressing	1 tbsp	75	7	86
Jalapeño peppers	1 tbsp	10	0	0
Kale	1 oz	15	0	0
Kidney beans	¼ cup	55	0	0
Lettuce	1 leaf	5	0	0
Macaroni salad	½ cup	150	9	54
Mozzarella	1 oz	90	7	70
Part skim	1 oz	70	5	64
Mushrooms	¼ cup	5	0	0
Oil	1 tbsp	120	14	100
Onions	¼ cup	10	0	0
Oranges	2 oz	25	0	0
Pasta salad	½ cup	180	9	45
Parmesan, grated	1 tbsp	25	2	78
Peaches	2 slices	15	0	0
Peas	1 oz	25	0	0
Pepper rings, pickled	1 tbsp	5	0	0
Pickle spear	1	10	0	0
Pineapple:				
Canned	3.5 oz	100	0	0
Fresh	1 slice	45	0	0
Potato salad	½ cup	150	9	54
Provolone	1 oz	90	7	70
Radishes	.5 oz	5	0	0
Ranch dressing	1 tbsp	80	8	90
Red cabbage	¼ cup	5	0	0
Red onions	3 rings	5	0	0

	AMOUNT	CALORIES	FAT-GRAMS	% FAT
Reduced-calorie dressing:				
Bacon-tomato	1 tbsp	45	4	80
Creamy cucumber	1 tbsp	50	5	90
Italian	1 tbsp	25	2	72
Thousand Island	1 tbsp	20	1	50
Sesame sticks	1 oz	150	10	60
Shredded imitation cheese	1 oz	90	6	60
Soynuts	1 oz	120	7	52
Strawberries	2 oz	20	0	0
Sunflower seeds w/ raisins	1 oz	130	10	69
Swiss cheese	1 oz	105	8	67
Three-bean salad	½ cup	155	8	41
Thousand Island dressing	1 tbsp	80	8	88
Tomatoes	1 oz	5	0	0
Turkey bits	2 oz	70	3	39
Turkey ham	¼ cup	50	2	36
Watermelon	2 pcs	20	0	0
Wine vinegar	1 tbsp	5	0	0

SALAD DRESSINGS

(Most ladles at salad bars hold 2 to 6 tablespoons of salad dressing.)

	AMOUNT	CALORIES	FAT-GRAMS	% FAT
Anchovy mayonnaise	2 tbsp	195	21	98
Bleu Lorraine dressing	2 tbsp	115	12	94
Blue cheese dressing	2 tbsp	149	16	97
Blue cheese French dressing	2 tbsp	185	20	98
Boiled dressing	2 tbsp	35	1	26
Buttermilk dressing	2 tbsp	50	3	55
Caesar dressing	2 tbsp	155	16	92

	AMOUNT	CALORIES	FAT-GRAMS	% FAT
Caper dressing	2 tbsp	190	21	99
Celery seed dressing	2 tbsp	225	21	84
Chiffonade French dressing	2 tbsp	170	19	99
Chive French dressing	2 tbsp	185	20	98
Creamy garlic dressing	2 tbsp	150	16	97
Creamy Italian dressing	2 tbsp	165	18	99
Chutney dressing	2 tbsp	185	20	98
Cocktail sauce	2 tbsp	35	0	0
Cream cheese grenadine	2 tbsp	90	5	50
Cucumber dressing	2 tbsp	90	10	100
Curry dressing	2 tbsp	205	22	97
Dijon dressing	2 tbsp	150	17	100
Dill weed dressing	2 tbsp	85	9	96
French dressing	2 tbsp	185	20	98
Fruit French dressing	2 tbsp	130	14	95
Garlic dressing	2 tbsp	155	17	99
Ginger dressing	2 tbsp	190	20	95
Ginger syrup	2 tbsp	90	0	0
Ginger vinaigrette	2 tbsp	170	18	94
Green Goddess dressing	2 tbsp	120	13	99
Guacamole dressing	2 tbsp	105	11	96
Honey fruit dressing	2 tbsp	50	3	55
Horseradish French dressing	2 tbsp	170	19	99
Hot bacon dressing	2 tbsp	235	15	57
Italian dressing	2 tbsp	145	14	86
Lemon ginger dressing	2 tbsp	85	7	75
Lemon syrup	2 tbsp	60	0	0
Lime syrup	2 tbsp	60	0	0
Louie sauce	2 tbsp	135	13	87
Mayonnaise	2 tbsp	200	22	98
Mustard mayonnaise	2 tbsp	155	17	97

	AMOUNT	CALORIES	FAT-GRAMS	% FAT
Oil & vinegar dressing	2 tbsp	140	14	90
Oil-free dressing	2 tbsp	15	0	0
Orange & poppy seed vinaigrette	2 tbsp	180	18	91
Orange & poppy seed oil-free dressing	2 tbsp	35	0	0
Orange syrup	2 tbsp	75	0	0
Peanut butter dressing	2 tbsp	200	21	95
Pesto dressing	2 tbsp	140	14	90
Ranch-style dressing	2 tbsp	160	16	90
Rémoulade dressing	2 tbsp	175	19	98
Roquefort dressing	2 tbsp	120	12	91
Russian dressing	2 tbsp	135	14	93
Sesame dressing	2 tbsp	180	16	80
Sesame seed dressing	2 tbsp	225	21	84
Shogun dressing	2 tbsp	125	13	94
Sun-dried tomato vinaigrette	2 tbsp	75	3	36
Tartar sauce	2 tbsp	160	17	96
Thousand Island dressing	2 tbsp	165	17	93
Low-calorie	2 tbsp	35	2	50
Tomato-basil vinaigrette, low-calorie	2 tbsp	10	0	0
Tomato French dressing	2 tbsp	80	7	80
Tropical fruit dressing	2 tbsp	110	11	90
Victor dressing	2 tbsp	95	10	98
Vinaigrette	2 tbsp	170	18	94
Walnut vinaigrette dressing	2 tbsp	130	14	95
Yogurt dressing	2 tbsp	35	2	50
Zero dressing (low-calorie)	2 tbsp	5	0	0

SANDWICHES

(Unless otherwise indicated, sandwiches are made with 2 slices of bread.)

	AMOUNT	CALORIES	FAT-GRAMS	% FAT
Bacon, lettuce & tomato sandwich	1	335	16	43
Bacon, lettuce, tomato & avocado sandwich	1	490	30	55
Bagel w/ cream cheese	1 bagel	325	17	47
Bagel w/ cream cheese & smoked salmon or lox	1 bagel	425	21	44
Beef:				
BBQ roast beef on bun (w/ BBQ sauce)	1	250	8	29
Beef pocket sandwich (beef, lettuce & tomato in pita)	1	270	5	17
Deluxe (roast beef, feta, lettuce, tomato, garlic, onion & olive oil in pita)	1	410	27	59

	AMOUNT	CALORIES	FAT-GRAMS	% FAT
Coney Island sandwich (grilled ground beef & frankfurter, mayo & mustard on triple-decker bun)	1	635	46	65
English pub beef (roast beef & horseradish dressing on Kaiser roll)	1	480	34	64
French dip	1	360	15	37
Hot roast beef sandwich w/ gravy	1	420	15	32
Italian beef (roast beef, peppers & onions on hoagie roll)	1	625	39	56
Italian meatball hero	1	535	25	42
Papa Joe's	1	280	11	35
Philly beef sandwich (roast beef, mushrooms, onions, melted cheese & dressing on French roll)	1	820	33	36
Roast beef sandwich (w/ lettuce & mayo)	1	430	26	54
Roast beef w/ cheese sandwich	1	440	27	55
Sloppy Joe	1	325	15	41
Steakball hero on French roll (3 meatballs)	1	470	22	43

	AMOUNT	CALORIES	FAT-GRAMS	% FAT
Bologna & cheese sandwich	1	425	28	59
Bologna sandwich (w/ mayo, lettuce & mustard)	1	405	19	42
Burgers:				
BBQ bacon burger (grilled beef, bacon, lettuce, tomato, cheese, mayonnaise & BBQ sauce on bun)	1	700	46	59
BBQ burger (grilled beef & BBQ sauce on bun)	1	440	22	45
BBQ chicken burger (grilled chicken, lettuce, tomato, onion & BBQ sauce on bun)	1	320	6	17
Deluxe (grilled chicken, lettuce, tomato, onion, BBQ sauce, cheese & mayo on bun)	1	495	22	40
Border chicken burger (grilled chicken, cheese, green chilies, tomatoes & guacamole on hard roll)	1	965	68	63

	AMOUNT	CALORIES	FAT-GRAMS	% FAT
Canadian bacon cheeseburger (grilled beef, cheese & Canadian bacon on bun)	1	570	34	53
Cheeseburger (grilled beef & cheese on bun)	1	485	30	55
Chicken cheeseburger (grilled chicken, cheese, lettuce, tomato & mayo on bun)	1	475	32	60
Chili guacamole burger (grilled beef, cheese, chili, tomatoes & guacamole on bun)	1	860	65	68
Deviled tuna cheeseburger (deviled tuna & cheese on bun)	1	405	24	53
French dip hamburger sandwich (grilled beef on French roll w/ au jus sauce)	1	410	20	44
w/ cheese		520	29	50
Grilled onion burger (grilled beef, lettuce, mayo & buttered grilled onions on bun)	1	565	38	60

	AMOUNT	CALORIES	FAT-GRAMS	% FAT
Guacamole burger (grilled beef, bacon, lettuce, tomato, mayo & guacamole on bun)	1	665	44	59
Hamburger (grilled beef, lettuce, tomato, pickle & onion on bun)	1	395	19	43
Mushroom burger (grilled beef & sautéed mushrooms on bun)	1	445	27	54
Patty melt (grilled beef & cheese on bread)	1	485	30	55
Peanut butter bacon burger (grilled beef, lettuce, tomato, mayo, bacon & peanut butter on bun)	1	765	53	62
Pizzaburger (grilled beef, mozzarella & pizza sauce on bun)	1	370	19	46
Refried bean burger (grilled beef, special sauce & refried beans on bun)	1	405	22	49

	AMOUNT	CALORIES	FAT-GRAMS	% FAT
Teriyaki burger (grilled ground beef, teriyaki sauce, cheese, tomato, lettuce, pineapple & mayo on bun)	1	635	41	58
Teriyaki chicken burger (chicken, teriyaki sauce, lettuce, tomato & onion on bun)	1	330	5	13
Turkey fillet burger deluxe (grilled turkey, bacon, tomato & cheese on bread)	1	445	25	50
Viennese schnitzelburger (grilled ground beef & fried egg on English muffin)	1	520	32	55
Cheese:				
French-fried cheese sandwich	1	590	33	50
Grilled cheese sandwich	1	360	23	57
w/ bacon		450	30	60
w/ chili		405	25	55
w/ ham		410	25	55
w/ olive		380	24	57
w/ tomato		370	23	56
Ham & cheese melt on hamburger bun	1	320	17	48

	AMOUNT	CALORIES	FAT-GRAMS	% FAT
Hot provolone sandwich	1	380	18	43
Chicken:				
Almond chicken salad sandwich	1	350	19	49
BBQ chicken burger (grilled chicken, lettuce, tomato, onion & BBQ sauce on bun)	1	320	6	17
Deluxe (grilled chicken, lettuce, tomato, onion, BBQ sauce, cheese & mayo on bun)	1	495	22	40
BBQ chicken sandwich deluxe (grilled chicken breast, BBQ sauce, cheese, lettuce, tomato & mayo on bun)	1	430	20	42
Border chicken burger (grilled chicken, cheese, green chilies, tomatoes & guacamole on hard roll)	1	965	68	63
Chicken-avocado sandwich	1	480	30	56
Chicken breast sandwich (w/ mayo & lettuce)	1	320	12	34

	AMOUNT	CALORIES	FAT GRAMS	% FAT
Chicken cheeseburger (grilled chicken, cheese, lettuce, tomato & mayo on bun)	1	475	32	60
Chicken club sandwich	1	545	26	43
Chicken mandarin salad sandwich (chicken salad & mandarin oranges on bread)	1	280	12	38
Chicken pocket sandwich (chicken, lettuce & tomato in pita)	1	255	3	10
Deluxe (chicken, lettuce, tomato, garlic, feta, onion & olive oil in pita)	1	395	25	57
Chicken salad sandwich	1	335	17	56
Chicken submarine (chicken, cheese, lettuce, tomato, avocado & dressing on French roll)	1	480	24	45
Teriyaki chicken burger (chicken, teriyaki sauce, lettuce, tomato & onion on bun)	1	330	5	13

	AMOUNT	CALORIES	FAT-GRAMS	% FAT
Coney Island sandwich (grilled ground beef & frankfurter, mayo & mustard on triple-decker bun)	1	635	46	65
Corn dog (4 oz)	1	330	20	55
Corned beef sandwich	1	370	19	46
Crabmeat salad sandwich	1	270	11	37
Cube steak sandwich (w/ onions, Swiss cheese & dressing on French bread)	1	505	21	37
Denver sandwich	1	350	19	49
Egg:				
Egg & bacon sandwich (w/ mayo)	1	503	32	57
Egg & cheese pocket sandwich (w/ sautéed onions, mushrooms & peppers in pita)	½ pita	365	21	52
Egg salad pocket sandwich (w/ lettuce & tomato in pita)	1	255	8	28
Egg salad sandwich	1	255	9	32
Ham & egg salad sandwich	1	305	15	44
Mexican egg sandwich (poached egg, cheese, tomatoes & refried beans on ½ English muffin)	1	230	13	51

	AMOUNT	CALORIES	FAT-GRAMS	% FAT
Tuna & egg salad sandwich	1	305	14	41
Welsh egg (egg salad, bacon, tomato & cheese on English muffin)	1	580	36	56
Fish sandwich (hot seafood, cheese & tomato on sourdough bread)	1	650	32	44
Frankfurters:				
BBQ frankfurter w/ bun	1	290	16	49
Coney Island sandwich (grilled ground beef & frankfurter, mayo & mustard on triple-decker bun)	1	635	46	65
Corn dog (4 oz)	1	330	20	55
Frankfurter & chili on bun	1	320	18	51
Frankfurter & sauerkraut on bun	1	280	16	52
Frankfurter, chili & cheese on bun	1	330	20	54
Frankfurter deluxe (frankfurter, relish, ketchup & mustard on bun)	1	310	16	46
Frankfurter w/ bacon & cheese on bun	1	370	24	58
Franks & baked beans on bun	1	360	17	43

	AMOUNT	CALORIES	FAT GRAMS	% FAT
Sloppy franks on bun	1	430	28	59
Stuffed BBQ frankfurter on bun (bread dressing)	1	340	19	50
French dip	1	360	15	37
Gyro	1	505	23	41
Ham & cheese sandwich (w/ lettuce & mayo)	1	410	23	50
Ham & egg salad sandwich	1	305	15	44
Ham & turkey salad sandwich	1	280	10	32
Ham salad sandwich	1	355	20	51
Ham sandwich (w/ lettuce & mayo)	1	365	19	47
Hot sandwiches:				
Hot chicken sandwich w/ 2 oz gravy	1	345	10	26
Hot pork sandwich w/ 2 oz gravy	1	420	18	38
Hot provolone sandwich	1	380	18	43
Hot roast beef sandwich w/ gravy	1	420	15	32
Hot turkey sandwich w/ 2 oz gravy	1	340	10	26
Pizza sandwich (French bread, cheese & pizza sauce)	1	375	23	55
Reuben sandwich	1	485	28	52
Turkey Divan on English muffin (w/ broccoli & Mornay sauce)	1	520	21	36

	AMOUNT	CALORIES	FAT-GRAMS	% FAT
Italian hoagie (salami, bologna, ham, cheese, tomato, onion, peppers, lettuce & dressing on hoagie roll)	1	490	27	49
Italian sausage sandwich (w/ peppers, onion & olive on Italian roll)	1	620	44	64
Knockwurst sandwich (w/ mustard on French roll)	1	875	65	67
Liverwurst sandwich	1	305	14	41
Lobster salad sandwich	1	270	11	36
Mexican egg sandwich (poached egg, cheese, tomatoes & refried beans on ½ English muffin)	1	230	13	51
Monte Cristo	1	405	22	49
Muffuletta sandwich	1	600	31	46
New York steak sandwich (grilled lean New York steak on French roll)	1	340	13	34
Oyster sandwich, fried	1	710	23	29
Peanut butter sandwiches:				
Peanut butter & jelly sandwich	1	360	19	48

	AMOUNT	CALORIES	FAT-GRAMS	% FAT
Peanut butter bacon burger (grilled ground beef, lettuce, tomato, mayo, bacon & peanut butter on bun)	1	765	53	62
Peanut butter sandwich	1	340	19	50
Sesame Street club sandwich (peanut butter, bacon, lettuce & tomato)	1	570	33	52
Philly beef sandwich (roast beef, onions, mushrooms, melted cheese & dressing on French roll)	1	820	33	36
Pocket sandwiches (in pita bread):				
Beef pocket sandwich (beef, lettuce & tomato)	1	270	5	17
Deluxe (roast beef, feta, lettuce, tomato, garlic, onion & olive oil)	1	410	27	59
Chicken pocket sandwich (chicken, lettuce & tomato)	1	255	3	10
Deluxe (chicken, lettuce, tomato, garlic, feta, onion & olive oil)	1	395	25	57

	AMOUNT	CALORIES	FAT-GRAMS	% FAT
Egg & cheese pocket sandwich (w/ sautéed onions, mushrooms & peppers)	½ pita	365	21	52
Egg salad pocket sandwich (w/ lettuce & tomato)	1	255	8	28
Veggie pocket sandwich (sprouts, onion, olives, tomatoes, mayo, lettuce & mushrooms)	1	340	18	47
w/ avocado		495	32	58
w/ avocado & cheese		610	41	61
w/ cheese		455	27	53
Polish sausage sandwich (w/ Swiss cheese & sauerkraut on bun)	1	565	41	65
Pork:				
BBQ pork (w/ BBQ sauce on French roll)	1	280	7	22
Hot pork sandwich w/ 2 oz gravy	1	420	18	38
Provolone sandwich, hot	1	380	18	43
Salami sandwich (2 oz salami, mayo & lettuce)	1	455	30	59
w/ 1 oz cheese		450	29	58
Salmon salad sandwich	1	275	12	39

	AMOUNT	CALORIES	FAT-GRAMS	% FAT
Seafood salad sandwich	1	280	11	36
Sesame Street club sandwich (peanut butter, bacon, lettuce & tomato)	1	570	33	52
Shrimp club sandwich	1	515	26	45
Shrimp croissant sandwich	1	365	24	59
Shrimp salad sandwich	1	290	14	43
Curried		295	14	43
Stromboli boats (spicy ground beef, & mozzarella on Kaiser roll)	1	330	17	46
Submarine sandwich (salami, pepperoni, summer sausage, provolone, mozzarella, Swiss cheese, mayo, mustard, lettuce & tomato on French roll)	1	540	29	48
Tuna:				
Deviled tuna cheeseburger (deviled tuna & cheese on bun)	1	405	24	53
Grilled tuna w/ cheese on rye	1	490	26	48
Tuna & egg salad sandwich	1	305	14	41
Tuna finger sandwiches	2 slices	290	14	43

SANDWICHES

	AMOUNT	CALORIES	FAT-GRAMS	% FAT
Tuna fish salad sandwich	1	310	14	40
Tuna patty sandwich (patty, cheese, lettuce, tomato & tartar sauce)	1	505	32	57
Tuna sandwich Italian-style (tuna salad, peppers, onion, pizza sauce & mozzarella on torpedo roll)	1	485	27	50
Turkey:				
Ham & turkey salad sandwich	1	280	10	32
Hot turkey sandwich w/ 2 oz gravy	1	340	10	26
Oriental turkey salad sandwich (diced turkey, celery, grapes, water chestnuts & mayo)	1	285	12	38
Turkey & cream cheese sandwich w/ cranberry chutney	1	470	28	54
Turkey Divan on English muffin (w/ broccoli & Mornay sauce)	1	520	21	36
Turkey fillet burger deluxe (grilled turkey, bacon, tomato & cheese on bread)	1	445	25	50

	AMOUNT	CALORIES	FAT-GRAMS	% FAT
Turkey sandwich (w/ lettuce & mayo)	1	315	12	34
Deluxe (w/ bacon, cheese, lettuce, tomato, & dressing on 1 slice bread)	1	475	24	45
Veggie-filled croissant sandwich w/ cheese	1	475	30	57
Veggie pocket sandwich (sprouts, onion, olives, tomatoes, mayo, lettuce & mushrooms in pita)	1	340	18	47
w/ avocado		495	32	58
w/ avocado & cheese		610	41	61
w/ cheese		455	27	53
Veggie sandwich (sprouts, onion, olives, tomatoes, lettuce, mayo & mushrooms)	1	340	19	50
w/ avocado		494	33	60
w/ avocado & cheese		610	42	62
w/ cheese		455	28	55
Viennese schnitzelburger (ground beef & fried egg on English muffin)	1	520	32	55
Welsh egg (egg salad, bacon, tomato & cheese on English muffin)	1	580	36	56

SAUCES & SPREADS

	AMOUNT	CALORIES	FAT-GRAMS	% FAT
A.1. Steak Sauce	1 tbsp	15	0	0
Aioli sauce	2 tbsp	195	21	98
Au jus	2 tbsp	55	6	96
Bacon sauce	¼ cup	185	14	69
Barbecue sauce	2 tbsp	15	0	0
Béarnaise sauce	¼ cup	220	22	89
Béchamel sauce	¼ cup	90	7	68
Bordelaise sauce	¼ cup	45	3	57
Brown sauce	¼ cup	20	0	0
Butter sauce	2 tbsp	205	23	100
Caper sauce	¼ cup	135	11	74
Cardinal sauce	¼ cup	95	7	66
Champagne sauce	¼ cup	115	40	79
Chateaubriand sauce	¼ cup	65	6	84
Cheese sauce	¼ cup	105	8	68
Cherry sauce	2 tbsp	25	0	0
Cocktail sauce	2 tbsp	35	0	0
Cranberry sauce	¼ cup	90	0	0
Cream sauce	¼ cup	80	6	66
Cucumber sauce	¼ cup	85	8	83
Cumberland sauce	2 tbsp	70	0	0

	AMOUNT	CALORIES	FAT-GRAMS	% FAT
Daikon (Chinese horseradish)	⅓ cup	15	0	0
Dijonnaise sauce	¼ cup	65	5	69
Duxelles sauce	¼ cup	80	6	69
Enchilada sauce	¼ cup	25	1	37
Gravy	¼ cup	80	6	67
Guacamole sauce	2 tbsp	40	4	88
Hollandaise sauce	2 tbsp	185	20	97
Horseradish sauce	¼ cup	65	4	56
Horseradish sour cream	2 tbsp	100	11	99
Ketchup	1 tbsp	20	0	0
Kirsch sauce	¼ cup	140	9	58
Lemon butter	2 tbsp	55	5	83
Lyonnaise sauce	¼ cup	45	2	38
Madeira sauce	¼ cup	30	1	28
Mayonnaise	1 tbsp	100	11	99
Meunière sauce	¼ cup	200	22	99
Milanaise sauce	¼ cup	65	4	54
Mock Hollandaise sauce	2 tbsp	95	9	85
Mornay sauce	¼ cup	100	7	62
Mousseline sauce	¼ cup	200	20	90
Mushroom sauce	¼ cup	90	6	60
Mustard	1 tbsp	5	0	0
Mustard sauce	¼ cup	95	6	58
Hot	1 tbsp	25	0	0
Oriental	1 tbsp	35	2	51
Newburg sauce	¼ cup	110	9	73
Orange sauce	¼ cup	105	0	0
Oyster sauce	¼ cup	110	7	58
Pesto	1 tbsp	155	15	86
Piquante sauce	¼ cup	25	0	0
Sabayon sauce	¼ cup	55	3	49

	AMOUNT	CALORIES	FAT-GRAMS	% FAT
Sour cream	1 tbsp	25	3	100
Sweet pickle relish	1 tbsp	20	0	0
Sweet-and-sour sauce	1 tbsp	30	0	0
Tabasco	¼ cup	0	0	0
Tartar sauce	1 tbsp	70	8	100
Teriyaki sauce	1 tbsp	30	0	0
Velouté sauce	¼ cup	65	5	67
Worcestershire sauce	1 tbsp	60	0	0

SEEFOOD

	AMOUNT	CALORIES	FAT-GRAMS	% FAT
Baked fish	5 oz	245	11	40
Bass:				
Bass fillet w/ sorrel & cream sauce	7 oz	390	21	48
Sea bass in champagne & butter sauce	8 oz	480	27	51
Sea bass w/ shrimp stuffing	8 oz	415	12	24
Bluefish cheese casserole	10 oz	455	22	43
Blackened fish	6.5 oz	390	20	46
Bouillabaisse	12 oz	235	9	35
Broiled fish	5 oz	245	11	40
Catfish:				
Blackened	6.5 oz	390	20	46
Breaded & fried	6 oz	400	24	54
Cioppino	12 oz	440	17	35
Clams:				
Breaded & fried clams	20 sm	380	21	50
Cherrystone clams	9 lg	135	2	13
Clams & chips (4 oz clams, 4 oz fries)	1 serving	650	28	39

	AMOUNT	CALORIES	FAT-GRAMS	% FAT
Clam fritters	3 oz	170	9	48
Deviled clam patties	4 oz	320	14	39
Fried clams	6 oz	380	20	47
Steamed clams (1 lb in shells)	20 sm	135	2	13
w/ fresh tomatoes, basil & garlic		265	8	28
w/ olive oil & lemon		335	21	56
Cod:				
Codfish cakes (2 oz each)	2	340	14	37
Dill smoked cod	5 oz	150	3	18
Fish & chips (4 oz cod, 4 oz fries)	1 serving	575	27	42
Scrod, breaded & fried	6 oz	400	24	54
Crab:				
Alaskan crab legs (6 oz)	1 leg	145	1	6
Crab in black bean sauce	½ crab	330	24	66
Crab cakes (2 oz each)	2	240	15	56
Crab Imperial	8 oz	450	32	64
Crabmeat au gratin	6 oz	285	16	50
Crabmeat & macaroni Newburg	8 oz	305	14	41
Crab Mornay (crab, mushrooms, cheese sauce, toast)	main dish	500	34	61

	AMOUNT	CALORIES	FAT-GRAMS	% FAT
Crab tostada (crab, beans, cheese, olives, avocado, sour cream)	1	920	47	46
Deviled crab	5 oz	225	13	52
Dungeness crab, cracked	½ of 2-lb crab	230	4	16
Dungeness crab in cream sauce (crab, asparagus, avocado, jack cheese)	1 crab	715	45	56
Fried soft-shell blue crab	1 lg	320	23	65
Herb-seasoned cracked crab	½ crab	240	14	53
Imitation crab	3 oz	85	1	10
King crabmeat soufflé (4" x 6")	1 serving	310	16	47
Crawfish étoufée (crawfish, rice)	8 oz	390	17	39
Deep-fat fried fish	4 oz	440	19	39
Fillets Florentine	4 oz	230	10	39
Fillets piccata	4 oz	300	22	66
Fillets w/ beer-cheese sauce	6 oz	600	42	63
Fish & chips (4 oz fish, 4 oz fries)	1 serving	575	27	42
Fish taco (fish, lettuce, 1 tbsp sour cream)	1	265	15	51
Fisherman's platter (5 pcs fish, 2.5 oz fries)	1 serving	730	40	49

	AMOUNT	CALORIES	FAT-GRAMS	% FAT
Flounder, stuffed				
w/ lobster	1 fillet	545	33	54
Haddock:				
Baked haddock in				
Newburg sauce	5 oz	400	21	47
Haddock fillet platter				
(w/ potatoes,				
tomatoes,				
mushrooms)	5 oz	875	54	56
Halibut:				
Broiled halibut	5 oz	245	11	40
Halibut w/ cream				
sherry sauce	5 oz	315	17	49
Halibut fillet				
Amandine	4 oz	255	17	60
À l'orange				
(5 oz fillet,				
2 oz sauce)	1 serving	320	12	34
Halibut steak,				
baked	5 oz	245	11	40
Lobster-stuffed				
halibut fillets w/				
Newburg sauce	8 oz	500	30	54
Pan-fried halibut				
(breaded)	5 oz	395	17	39
Poached halibut	5 oz	180	4	20
Herring:				
Kippered (1 med pc)	1.4 oz	85	5	53
Pickled	½ oz	40	3	67
Lobster:				
Boiled or steamed				
lobster	1.25 lb	110	1	8
Broiled lobster tail				
beurre	8 oz	335	16	45

	AMOUNT	CALORIES	FAT-GRAMS	% FAT
Crumb-topped lobster tails	1 tail	170	7	37
Lobster w/ crab stuffing & creamy cheese sauce	1 lobster	695	49	63
Lobster Newburg (w/o rice)	6 oz	70	3	37
w/ 1 popover		320	17	48
Lobster-stuffed halibut fillets w/ Newburg sauce	8 oz	500	30	54
Lobster Thermidor	5 oz ramekin	190	10	47
Mixed seafood grill	4 oz	280	9	29
Mussels:				
Mussels & clams, steamed in wine & garlic (½ lb in shells)	1 serving	205	5	23
Mussels marinara	½ lb	210	8	34
Steamed mussels in olive oil, garlic & tomatoes	1 doz	330	12	33
Orange roughy, grilled	5 oz	210	10	43
Pan-fried fish	5 oz	395	17	39
Poached fish	5 oz	180	4	20
Portuguese fish stew	12 oz	475	21	40
Oysters:				
Fried oysters	3 lg	200	11	49
Oysters au gratin	8 oz	295	18	55
Oysters Rockefeller	3 oysters	80	5	58

	AMOUNT	CALORIES	FAT-GRAMS	% FAT
Oysters topped w/ bacon, crab & Newburg sauce	6 oysters	280	14	45
Raw oysters	6 med	70	2	26
Scalloped oysters	8 oz	400	20	45
Redfish:				
Blackened redfish	3.5 oz	195	11	51
Cajun redfish	3.5 oz	195	11	51
Red mullet Triestina (fish, wine, lemon juice, capers, fried bread)	8 oz	475	17	32
Red snapper Liguria (fish, tomato, wine sauce, anchovies	8 oz	405	12	26
Rockfish amandine	8 oz	565	35	56
Salmon:				
Alder-smoked salmon	6 oz	265	16	54
BBQ salmon	6 oz	265	16	54
Hickory-smoked salmon	6 oz	265	16	54
Poached salmon	8 oz	265	8	27
Salmon cake	3.5 oz	240	15	56
Salmon croquettes	4 oz	370	19	46
Salmon coulibiac (fish, rice, puff pastry)	1 serving	1,640	108	59
Salmon in crust	12 oz	915	48	47
Salmon loaf	5 oz	205	9	40
Salmon, noodles & mushroom casserole	12 oz	595	32	48
Salmon quiche (crustless)	1/6 of 9" quiche	280	17	55

	AMOUNT	CALORIES	FAT-GRAMS	% FAT
Salmon shortcake (creamed salmon, 1 biscuit)	1 serving	495	28	51
Salmon teriyaki	6 oz	260	6	21
Salmon topped w/ guacamole sauce & sour cream	6 oz	635	46	65
Scalloped salmon	5 oz	205	9	40
Smoked salmon	3 oz	100	4	36
Stuffed salmon (garden vegetable stuffing)	6 oz	330	20	54
Scallops:				
Broiled scallops w/ ginger soy sauce	5 oz	155	6	35
Coquilles St. Jacques	5-oz ramekin	220	10	41
Imitation scallops	3 oz	85	0	0
Scallops & prawns w/ risotto	9 oz	445	5	10
Scallops Dijonnaise	4 oz	215	11	46
Scallops en brochette	1 brochette	290	7	22
Scallops in garlic butter	5 oz	270	16	53
Scallops w/ fettuccine in cream sauce	10 oz	1,000	61	55
Scrod, breaded & fried	6 oz	400	24	54
Seafood à la meunière (seafood fillets, white sauce)	5 oz	445	33	67
Seafood, breaded & fried	6 oz	400	24	54

SEAFOOD

	AMOUNT	CALORIES	FAT-GRAMS	% FAT
Seafood brochette	1 brochette	170	3	16
Seafood cakes	4 oz	340	14	37
Seafood fillets amandine	4 oz	255	17	60
Seafood in cream sauce	5 oz	315	17	49
Seafood, meat & vegetable chow mein:				
w/ pan-fried noodles	main dish	680	36	48
w/ soft noodles	12 oz	565	30	48
Seafood Medley (shrimp, scallops, prawns, halibut, Cajun sauce)	4 oz	360	14	35
Seafood pot pie	1	555	31	50
Seafood risotto	9 oz	445	5	10
Shark teriyaki	4 oz	140	5	32
Shellfish:				
Imitation shellfish (surimi)	3 oz	85	1	11
Shellfish Medley w/ aioli sauce (clams, mussels, crab, shrimp)	8 oz	355	6	15
Shrimp:				
Bahía shrimp stir-fry	8 oz	305	19	56
Baked stuffed prawns	6 prawns	340	19	50
BBQ shrimp	6 oz	255	2	70
Beer-batter shrimp	6 oz	410	26	57
Boiled shrimp	5 oz	155	2	12
Butterflied shrimp teriyaki	6 oz	255	1	35
Cajun shrimp	6 oz	255	2	70
Cajun shrimp kabobs	1 kabob	221	8	32

	AMOUNT	CALORIES	FAT-GRAMS	% FAT
Chinese fried shrimp	6 oz	535	28	47
French-fried breaded shrimp	6 oz	410	26	57
Grilled prawns w/ tomato & basil	3 prawns	270	16	54
Hong Kong shrimp (⅔ cup shrimp, vegetables, 1 cup rice)	1 serving	640	8	11
Imitation shrimp	3 oz	85	1	10
Peel & eat shrimp	5 oz	155	2	12
Phoenix-tail shrimp	4 oz	305	12	36
per 1 tbsp dipping sauce	*add*	29	0	0
Prawns & scallops in lemon cream sauce	5 oz	375	18	43
Princess prawns (fried prawns, cashews, hot sauce)	8 oz	505	25	44
Shrimp & noodles au gratin	6 oz	265	12	41
Shrimp Calypso (shrimp, butter, brandy, tomato sauce)	8 oz	415	26	56
Shrimp chimichanga (shrimp, cheese, tortilla, sour cream)	1 serving	595	35	53
Shrimp chow mein (w/o noodles)	1 cup	220	10	41
Shrimp Creole	8 oz	300	9	27

	AMOUNT	CALORIES	FAT-GRAMS	% FAT
Shrimp curry				
(w/o rice)	6 oz	235	14	53
Shrimp De Jonghe	6 shrimp	340	19	50
Shrimp enchilada				
(w/o topping)	1	370	21	51
Shrimp fried rice	8 oz	320	10	28
Shrimp jambalaya				
(shrimp, rice,				
ham, peppers,				
tomato sauce)	8 oz	290	8	25
Shrimp rice casserole				
(2 oz shrimp,				
1½ cups rice,				
sauce)	1 serving	360	13	33
Shrimp scampi	3 oz	230	16	63
w/ saffron rice	6 shrimp	825	49	53
Shrimp Siciliano				
(shrimp, tomato,				
red wine sauce)	8 oz	415	26	56
Shrimp tostada				
(beans, cheese,				
olives, avocado,				
sour cream)	1	940	47	45
Shrimp w/ bean curd				
& vegetables	12 oz	520	21	36
Shrimp w/ garlic				
butter	4 oz	320	27	76
Shrimp w/ lobster				
sauce	4 oz	345	16	42
Shrimp w/ peppers	4 oz	165	5	27
Sizzling rice shrimp	8 oz	460	19	37
Stir-fried shrimp:				
w/ snow peas	8 oz	245	12	44
w/ vegetables	8 oz	245	18	66

	AMOUNT	CALORIES	FAT-GRAMS	% FAT
Sweet-and-sour shrimp	6 oz	235	12	46
Sizzling sweet-and-sour seafood	8 oz	460	19	37
Sole:				
Broccoli-stuffed sole	4 oz	460	25	49
Fillet of sole, Florentine	6 oz	365	15	37
Sole à la Bonne Femme (sole, mushrooms, cream sauce)	6 oz	415	18	39
Sole in sweet-and-sour sauce	4 oz	460	29	57
Sole le Marmère (breaded & fried sole)	6 oz	605	37	55
Sole w/ shrimp, crab & mushroom stuffing	5 oz	340	15	39
Squid:				
Calamari Milanese (squid, egg batter, white wine, capers, lemon)	3 oz	190	11	52
Calamari w/ linguine (squid, linguine, tomato sauce, clams)	1.5 cup	410	6	13
Fried squid	5 oz	248	11	40
Squid & snow peas stir-fry w/ noodles	main dish	475	19	36

	AMOUNT	CALORIES	FAT-GRAMS	% FAT
Squid & vegetable stir-fry	main dish	215	11	46
Stir-fried calamari	5 oz	248	11	40
Stuffed squid	8 oz	285	10	31
Sturgeon, smoked	3 oz	145	4	24
Sweet-and-sour seafood kabob	1	205	5	22
Swordfish:				
Broiled swordfish steak (fish, olive oil, garlic, lemon)	8 oz	600	45	68
Grilled swordfish steak puttanesca (fish, capers, calamata olives)	5 oz	410	32	70
Marinated grilled swordfish steak	4 oz	180	10	50
Swordfish kabob	1	150	7	42
Tempura fish fillet	1	440	21	51
Trout:				
Grilled rainbow trout	4 oz	245	12	44
Stuffed trout (⅓ cup bread stuffing)	1 trout	595	40	60
w/ Swiss chard		395	30	68
Trout sauté amandine	4	235	12	46
Tuna:				
Creamed tuna w/ peas	6 oz	240	11	41
Grilled tuna	4 oz	180	8	39
w/ fresh tomato & basil sauce		345	21	55
Mandarin tuna (tuna, rice, noodles, vegetables, sauce)	8 oz	520	17	29

	AMOUNT	CALORIES	FAT-GRAMS	% FAT
Scalloped tuna	5 oz	205	9	40
Tuna à la king	6 oz	275	11	36
Tuna & celery on biscuits	3 oz	305	15	44
Tuna fish turnover	1	375	23	55
Tuna Florentine	8 oz	520	42	72
Tuna loaf	5 oz	355	24	61
Tuna noodle casserole	8 oz	300	12	36
Tuna rarebit	8 oz	315	17	48
Tuna rice casserole	8 oz	210	8	34
Tuna tetrazzini	8 oz	505	18	32
Whitefish:				
Broiled whitefish amandine	8 oz	655	49	67
Mediterranean whitefish (fish, olive oil, lemon, onions)	8 oz	260	8	27
Smoked whitefish	3 oz	90	1	10
Whitefish stuffed w/ wild rice	8 oz	428	17	36

SEAFOOD

SOUPS

	AMOUNT	CALORIES	FAT-GRAMS	% FAT
Avgolemono soup (Greek)	8 oz	185	5	24
Barley soups:				
Barley & mushroom soup	8 oz	180	7	35
Cream of barley w/ prosciutto	10 oz	340	20	53
Scotch barley	6 oz	75	2	24
Bean soup	8 oz	185	5	24
Bisques:				
Clam	6 oz	240	16	59
Oyster	6 oz	330	15	57
Shrimp	6 oz	175	13	67
Black bean soup	8 oz	190	5	23
Beef broth	8 oz	20	1	45
Beef Calcutta (beef stock, beef, vegetables, rice, curry, apple)	6 oz	105	5	43
Beef consommé	8 oz	30	0	0
Beef noodle soup	6 oz	55	1	16
Beef rice soup	6 oz	55	1	16
Beef soup w/ farina dumpling	8 oz	65	3	42

	AMOUNT	CALORIES	FAT-GRAMS	% FAT
Blueberry soup				
(w/ cream)	8 oz	125	6	43
Borscht (2 tbsp sour				
cream)	8 oz	90	6	59
Polish-style (w/ duck				
& sausage)	8 oz	110	8	67
Bouillabaisse (French)	10 oz	235	9	35
Cabbage soups:				
Old-fashioned				
cabbage soup	8 oz	165	10	54
Sauerkraut soup	8 oz	175	14	72
Viennese cabbage				
soup (w/ Polish				
sausage)	8 oz	240	20	75
Cajun Creole soup	6 oz	75	1	12
Cheddar cheese soup	6 oz	170	11	57
Chicken Acapulco				
(chicken broth,				
chicken, avocado,				
tortilla, cheese)	8 oz	280	13	41
Chicken broth	8 oz	35	1	26
Chicken consommé	8 oz	30	0	0
Chicken Calcutta				
(chicken, stock,				
vegetables, rice,				
curry, apple)	6 oz	105	5	43
Chicken corn chowder	8 oz	115	6	46
Chicken giblets w/ rice	6 oz	80	4	45
Chicken gumbo	8 oz	125	5	36
Chicken mulligatawny	6 oz	110	6	48
Chicken noodle soup	6 oz	80	2	22
Chicken vegetable				
soup	6 oz	65	1	14
Chili	6 oz	150	4	24

	AMOUNT	CALORIES	FAT-GRAMS	% FAT
Clam bisque	6 oz	240	16	59
Chowders:				
Chicken corn chowder	8 oz	115	6	46
Clam chowder				
Boston	6 oz	140	7	46
Manhattan	6 oz	130	6	41
New England	6 oz	225	12	48
Corn chowder	6 oz	235	11	42
Crab chowder	6 oz	110	5	40
Fish chowder	6 oz	100	5	44
Potato chowder	6 oz	150	7	41
Turkey chowder	8 oz	125	3	22
Vegetable chowder	6 oz	85	5	52
Cioppino	12 oz	440	17	35
Cock-a-leekie	8 oz	185	4	20
Continental bean w/ bacon soup	6 oz	330	22	60
Corn chowder	6 oz	235	11	42
Country vegetable soup	6 oz	60	0	0
Crab chowder	6 oz	110	5	40
Crab gumbo	8 oz	105	4	34
Cream soups:				
Cream of almond soup	6 oz	205	16	70
Cream of asparagus soup	8 oz	170	10	53
Cream of broccoli soup	8 oz	155	11	64
Cream of carrot	6 oz	265	17	57
Cream of celery	6 oz	235	16	61
Cream of chicken	6 oz	245	15	55
Cream of mushroom	6 oz	280	19	61
Cream of oyster	8 oz	160	7	40

	AMOUNT	CALORIES	FAT-GRAMS	% FAT
Cream of spinach	6 oz	215	14	59
Cream of tomato	6 oz	170	9	48
Cream of vegetable	6 oz	195	11	51
Duchess	6 oz	225	14	56
Duchess cream of tomato	6 oz	155	8	46
Duck soup Parisienne	8 oz	20	1	41
Dutch vegetable soup	6 oz	170	10	53
Egg drop soup	6 oz	70	4	51
Fish chowder	6 oz	100	5	44
French onion soup	8 oz	385	25	58
Gazpacho	8 oz	60	2	30
Genovese fish soup	8 oz	480	20	37
Goulash soup (Hungarian)	8 oz	215	10	42
Guacamole soup	4 oz	115	9	70
Gumbos:				
Chicken	8 oz	125	5	36
Crab	8 oz	105	4	34
Shrimp	8 oz	105	4	34
Turkey	8 oz	95	4	38
Hot-and-sour soup	8 oz	75	2	24
Jellied chicken consommé	6 oz	40	1	21
Jellied tomato madrilene	6 oz	40	0	0
Lamb broth Anglaise	8 oz	115	5	39
Lentil soup (Polish)	6 oz	300	19	57
Lima bean & bacon soup	6 oz	280	21	68
Manhattan clam chowder	6 oz	130	6	41
Minestrone Italiano	6 oz	155	4	23
Minestrone w/ pesto	8 oz	220	7	29
Miso soup	8 oz	50	1	18

	AMOUNT	CALORIES	FAT-GRAMS	% FAT
Navy bean soup	8 oz	185	5	24
New England clam chowder	6 oz	225	12	48
Old-fashioned cabbage soup	8 oz	165	10	54
Olla podrida (black-eyed peas, rice, chorizo, sausage, chicken, ham, garbanzo beans, chicken stock)	8 oz	175	14	72
Onion soup	6 oz	95	5	47
Oxtail soup	8 oz	170	8	42
Oxtail soup à l'Anglaise	8 oz	125	5	35
Oyster bisque	6 oz	240	15	57
Oyster stew	8 oz	220	12	49
Pea soup:				
Green pea	8 oz	133	2	13
Split	8 oz	200	3	13
Philadelphia pepper pot	6 oz	125	6	43
Polish lentil soup	6 oz	300	19	57
Potato & leek soup	6 oz	195	12	55
Potato chowder	6 oz	150	7	41
Pot-au-feu	8 oz	135	5	33
Purée Mongol	6 oz	280	18	58
Raspberry creme (cold)	6 oz	100	1	9
Rice soup Florentine	8 oz	130	6	41
Sauerkraut soup	8 oz	175	14	72
Sausage & vegetable soup	8 oz	365	21	52
Shark fin soup	8 oz	195	5	23
Shrimp bisque	6 oz	175	13	67
Shrimp gumbo	8 oz	105	4	34
Sizzling rice soup	8 oz	170	5	26

	AMOUNT	CALORIES	FAT-GRAMS	% FAT
Sopa Royale (chicken stock, sherry, pimento, chicken, eggs, ham)	8 oz	100	4	36
Snapper soup	6 oz	230	9	35
Split-pea soup	6 oz	350	18	46
Stracciatella (egg & cheese soup)	8 oz	65	3	42
Tomato bouillon w/ rice	8 oz	65	1	14
Tomato rice soup	6 oz	135	5	33
Tortellini chicken soup	10 oz	310	10	29
Tortellini vegetable soup	10 oz	300	8	24
Turkey chowder	8 oz	125	3	22
Turkey Creole soup	8 oz	85	5	53
Turkey gumbo	8 oz	95	4	38
Turkish cucumber Iman	8 oz	130	8	56
Turtle soup (clear)	8 oz	60	0	0
Tuscan tomato soup (basil, tomato soup, toasted bread, olive oil)	8 oz	295	14	43
Vegetable chowder	6 oz	85	5	52
Vegetable, pasta & bean soup	10 oz	310	8	23
Vichyssoise	8 oz	165	15	82
Viennese cabbage soup (w/ Polish sausage)	8 oz	240	20	75
Wonton soup	8 oz	195	11	51
Zupp'alla Roma (escarole & cheese soup)	8 oz	115	7	54

SOUPS

VEGETABLES

(It may be assumed that most vegetables served in restaurants are cooked and/or served with a dollop or pat of butter.)

	AMOUNT	CALORIES	FAT-GRAMS	% FAT
Artichokes:				
Artichoke hearts sauté	3 oz	100	8	72
Artichokes au gratin	3 oz	150	7	42
Artichoke w/ butter sauce	1	265	23	78
Herbed Jerusalem artichokes	3 oz	130	12	83
Asparagus:				
Boiled/steamed asparagus, buttered	2.5 oz	35	2	53
Asparagus casserole	6 oz	165	10	54
Asparagus Dijon	4 oz	120	10	76
Asparagus-tomato stir-fry	3 oz	75	4	49
Lemon-buttered asparagus	3 oz	40	2	45
Bavarian cabbage	½ cup	115	7	55

	AMOUNT	CALORIES	FAT-GRAMS	% FAT
Beans & legumes:				
Baked beans	1 cup	240	2	7
Bean stew (kidney beans, tomatoes, onions, peppers)	3 oz	105	3	25
Black beans	1 cup	235	2	8
Black beans & rice (no fat added)	8 oz	315	1	3
Black-eyed peas	4 oz	140	2	13
Boston baked beans	1 cup	345	10	26
Bruna boner (Swedish beans)	4 oz	210	2	8
Chili:				
Beef chili verde	8 oz	270	15	50
Chili con carne	8 oz	350	21	54
Chili w/ macaroni	8 oz	255	6	21
Chili Sante Fe				
Beef	10 oz	340	17	45
Lamb	6 oz	260	13	45
Mexican pork chili	8 oz	590	41	63
San Antone chili	8 oz	590	41	63
Taos chili verde	8 oz	270	15	50
Gaucho beans (pinto beans, ground beef, bacon, tomatoes, seasoning)	8 oz	315	12	34
Green beans amandine	3 oz	85	6	63
Green beans & mushrooms (no fat added)	3 oz	25	0	0
Green beans & water chestnuts	3 oz	65	4	57
Green beans w/ butter & horseradish	3 oz	100	8	72

	AMOUNT	CALORIES	FAT-GRAMS	% FAT
Green beans Creole	3 oz	35	2	51
Green beans Lyonnaise	3 oz	60	4	62
Homestyle wax beans	3 oz	70	2	26
Lima beans & corn in cream	3 oz	100	4	36
Lima beans Creole (no fat added)	3 oz	60	0	0
Lima beans w/ onions	3 oz	145	4	25
Mexican bean stew	3 oz	105	3	25
Mexican red beans w/ pork	3 oz	320	19	53
Pasta e fagioli (pasta & beans)	1 cup	300	8	24
Pinto beans	1 cup	240	2	7
Pork & lima beans	1 cup	275	9	29
Red beans & rice w/ meat	8 oz	550	19	31
w/o meat	8 oz	315	1	3
Refried beans	½ cup	130	2	14
Shell beans w/ onions	1 cup	65	4	54
Southern green beans	3 oz	35	1	25
Spanish lima beans	1 cup	345	11	28
Succotash (lima beans, corn, tomato, bacon)	3 oz	95	3	28
w/ cream		155	6	35
Wax beans in bacon sauce	3 oz	65	3	43
Beets:				
Fresh beets, buttered	3 oz	45	2	42
Harvest beets	3 oz	80	2	22
Hot spiced beets	3 oz	85	2	21
Orange-glazed beets	3 oz	70	2	25

	AMOUNT	CALORIES	FAT-GRAMS	% FAT
Bok choy:				
Au gratin	3 oz	130	9	62
Oriental-style	3 oz	60	4	58
Broccoli:				
Broccoli, buttered	3 oz	40	2	43
Broccoli-carrot stir-fry	3 oz	95	6	56
Broccoli Mornay	4 oz	215	15	63
Broccoli Oriental	3 oz	140	8	52
Broccoli soufflé	4 oz	190	13	62
Broccoli w/ cheese	3 oz	190	14	66
French-fried broccoli	3 oz	260	16	55
Brussels sprouts:				
Brussels sprouts, buttered	3 oz	45	2	39
Brussels sprouts in onion cream	3 oz	105	8	69
Brussels sprouts Polonaise	3 oz	205	23	53
Cabbage:				
Bavarian cabbage	½ cup	115	7	55
Cabbage strudel	1	225	18	72
Chinese fried cabbage	3 oz	75	5	60
Colcannon (Irish cabbage)	6 oz	205	9	40
Country-style cabbage	½ cup	115	8	62
Dutch cabbage	3 oz	35	2	49
Escalloped cabbage	3 oz	65	3	40
Sauerkraut	3 oz	70	2	26
Sautéed cabbage	½ cup	90	8	79

	AMOUNT	CALORIES	FAT-GRAMS	% FAT
Carrots:				
Broccoli-carrot stir-fry	3 oz	95	6	56
Carrots & celery, buttered	3 oz	50	2	36
Carrots Lyonnaise	3 oz	65	3	43
Glazed carrots	3 oz	115	6	46
Peas & carrots	3 oz	85	2	22
Steamed carrots, buttered	3 oz	55	2	32
Turkish carrots	3 oz	175	8	41
Cauliflower:				
Au gratin	4 oz	110	7	57
Parmesan	3 oz	75	3	35
Celery:				
Braised celery	2.5 oz	30	2	58
Carrots & celery, buttered	3 oz	50	2	36
Peas & celery, buttered	3 oz	70	2	25
Chinese greens & bean curd in peanut sauce	10 oz	365	19	47
Colach (squash Mexican-style)	6 oz	200	10	45
Colcannon (Irish cabbage)	6 oz	205	9	40
Corn:				
Corn on the cob, buttered	1 ear	120	5	37
Corn pudding	4 oz	135	5	34
Lima beans & corn in cream	3 oz	100	4	36

	AMOUNT	CALORIES	FAT-GRAMS	% FAT
Mexican corn	3 oz	85	2	21
Succotash	3 oz	95	3	28
Crookneck squash soufflé	4 oz	70	4	51
Cucumbers in cream	3 oz	180	18	90
Delmonico potatoes	4 oz	105	3	25
Duchess potatoes	3 oz	155	9	52
Dutch cabbage	3 oz	35	2	49
Eggplant:				
Eggplant Creole	4 oz	40	1	23
Eggplant Lombardi	8 oz	280	11	35
Eggplant Parmigiana	8 oz	380	16	38
Eggplant w/ sherried mushrooms	3 slices	215	6	25
Fresh greens w/ bacon drippings	3 oz	90	7	71
Glazed parsnips	3 oz	145	6	37
Grilled vegetables	1 serving	240	21	78
Hong Kong spinach	3 oz	70	6	62
Kartoffel Klosse	3 balls	390	16	37
Lima beans & corn in cream	3 oz	100	4	36
Lima beans Creole	3 oz	60	0	0
Lima beans w/ onions	3 oz	145	4	25
Lyonnaise potatoes	4 oz	185	7	34
Mexican bean stew	3 oz	105	3	25
Mexican corn	3 oz	85	2	21
Mexican red beans w/ pork	3 oz	320	19	53
Moravian cabbage	4 oz	190	8	37
Mushrooms:				
Broiled fresh mushrooms	3 oz	50	4	70
Sautéed mushrooms	3 oz	45	4	78

	AMOUNT	CALORIES	FAT-GRAMS	% FAT
O'Brien potatoes	4 oz	165	7	38
Onions:				
Fried onion rings	1 med onion	550	47	77
Fried onions	2 oz	85	7	75
Glazed onions	3 oz	115	6	46
Pearl onions in cream sauce	3 oz	150	11	65
Pearl onions, Sarasota	3 oz	85	5	53
Orange-glazed beets	3 oz	70	2	25
Orange-glazed sweet potatoes (no fat added)	3.5 oz	130	0	0
Parsnips, glazed	3 oz	145	6	37
Peas:				
Green peas, buttered	3 oz	80	5	55
Peas & carrots	3 oz	85	2	22
Peas & celery, buttered	3 oz	70	2	25
Peas & mushrooms, buttered	3 oz	65	1	14
Peas & onions, buttered	3 oz	75	2	25
Peas & turnips, buttered	3 oz	95	5	48
Stir-fried Chinese pea pods & pepper	3 oz	115	7	55
Peppers:				
Sicilian fried peppers	2 oz	70	5	66
Stir-fried peppers	4 oz	165	13	71

	AMOUNT	CALORIES	FAT-GRAMS	% FAT
Pinto beans	1 cup	240	2	7
Pork & lima beans	1 cup	275	9	29
Potatoes:				
Baked potato	1 lg	270	0	0
w/ 1 oz bacon		350	6	15
w/ 1 oz bacon,				
¼ cup sour				
cream & chives		480	16	30
w/ 1 tbsp butter		370	11	27
w/ butter, bacon,				
sour cream, chives	580	22	34	
w/ cheese & bacon		760	26	31
w/ cheese &				
broccoli		760	26	31
w/ chili & cheese		700	23	29
w/ ¼ cup sour cream		400	11	24
Baked potato skins				
w/ cheese	¼ potato	60	3	29
Boiled potatoes,				
buttered	4 oz	125	3	22
Cottage-fries	4 oz	185	7	34
Creamed potatoes	4 oz	105	2	17
Delmonico potatoes	4 oz	105	3	25
Duchess potatoes	3 oz	155	9	52
Escalloped potatoes	4 oz	115	3	23
French fries	1 potato	215	11	46
Fried potato skins	¼ potato	55	3	50
Hash browns	½ cup	163	11	61
Home-fried potatoes	4 oz	220	8	33
Hot potato salad	1 cup	250	16	58
Kartoffel Klosse	3 balls	390	16	37
Lyonnaise potatoes	4 oz	185	7	34
Mashed or whipped				
potatoes	½ cup	125	3	29

	AMOUNT	CALORIES	FAT-GRAMS	% FAT
O'Brien potatoes	4 oz	165	7	38
Oven-roasted potatoes	1 med potato	210	11	47
Potato cake Parmesan	4 oz	170	7	37
Potato chips	1 oz	150	9	60
Chef-prepared	1 potato	285	14	44
Potato dumplings	2	145	1	6
Potatoes au gratin	4 oz	200	11	49
Potatoes Champs Élysées	9 oz	350	20	51
Potatoes Hongroise	6 oz	140	4	26
Potatoes Lorette	7 oz	685	45	59
Potatoes Theresa	8 oz	170	3	16
Potato gnocchi	5 oz	210	6	26
Potato pancakes	1 cake	495	13	24
Potato patty	1	255	16	56
Potato puffs	2	165	5	27
Potato slices (skin on)	1 potato	240	14	52
Potato wedges (skin on)	1 potato	240	14	52
Rissole potatoes	4 oz	200	11	49
Seasoned/coated fries	1 potato	305	12	35
Shoestring potatoes	1 potato	285	14	44
Spiral fries	1 potato	285	14	44
Stuffed potato	1 sm	180	5	25
Sweet potatoes. *See* separate entry.				
Ratatouille	8 oz	145	10	62
Rutabagas, buttered	3 oz	50	2	36
Sauerkraut	3 oz	70	2	26
Spinach:				
Hong Kong spinach (sautéed spinach, Oriental soy sauce)	3 oz	70	5	62

	AMOUNT	CALORIES	FAT-GRAMS	% FAT
Spinach w/ bacon drippings	3 oz	90	7	71
Spinach, buttered	3 oz	55	2	33
Spinach soufflé	4 oz	145	9	57
Wilted spinach	3 oz	130	11	76
Squash:				
Baked acorn squash	½ squash	165	4	22
Baked crookneck squash	3 oz	20	1	50
Baked squash (butter, brown sugar)	1 pc	75	4	47
Colach (squash Mexican-style)	6 oz	200	10	45
Crookneck squash, buttered	3 oz	35	2	51
Fresh okra, buttered	2.5 oz	50	3	52
Whipped fresh winter squash	3.5 oz	80	2	22
Zucchini à la Française	5 oz	120	6	45
Zucchini & tomatoes	½ cup	40	2	43
Zucchini fritters	2 each	76	6	71
Zucchini Neapolitan	4 oz	140	12	76
Shell beans w/ onions	1 cup	65	4	54
Sicilian fried peppers	2 oz	70	5	66
Spanish lima beans	1 cup	345	11	28
Stewed tomatoes	½ cup	55	2	31
Succotash	3 oz	95	3	28
Sweet potatoes:				
Candied sweet potatoes	3.5 oz	205	2	9
Escalloped sweet potato & apple	4 oz	145	3	19

VEGETABLES

	AMOUNT	CALORIES	FAT-GRAMS	% FAT
Mashed or whipped sweet potato	½ cup	135	4	26
Orange-glazed sweet potatoes	3.5 oz	130	0	0
Sweet potatoes w/ pecans	3.5 oz	240	5	19
Tomatoes:				
Baked or broiled tomatoes	3 oz	30	1	31
Baked stuffed tomato	1	55	1	16
Escalloped tomatoes	½ cup	115	5	39
Pan-fried tomatoes	4 oz	290	21	65
Stewed tomatoes	½ cup	55	2	31
Tomatoes & celery	½ cup	30	0	0
Tomatoes & okra	½ cup	55	2	33
Turkish carrots	3 oz	175	8	41
Turnips, buttered	3 oz	10	0	0
Turnips, Swedish-style	4 oz	190	10	47
Wax beans in bacon sauce	3 oz	65	3	43
Vegetable Medley	8 oz	100	4	35
Vegetables, creamed	3 oz	60	2	30
Vegetables amandine	3 oz	60	3	43
Vegetables au gratin	3 oz	90	6	59
Vegetables Hollandaise	4 oz	215	21	88
Vegetables Macedoine	3 oz	80	4	45
Vegetables Oriental	3 oz	35	3	82
Vegetable stir-fry w/ bean curd	8 oz	180	13	65
Zucchini à la Française	5 oz	120	6	45
Zucchini & tomatoes	½ cup	40	2	43
Zucchini fritters	2	75	6	72
Zucchini Neapolitan	4 oz	140	12	76

VEGETARIAN ENTRÉES

	AMOUNT	CALORIES	FAT-GRAMS	% FAT
Asparagus				
à la Polonaise				
(asparagus, egg,				
cream sauce,				
buttered crumbs)	8 oz	205	11	48
Avocado burgers:				
w/ bun	8 oz	565	30	48
w/o bun	8 oz	435	28	58
Bean burgers:				
w/ bun	8 oz	700	42	54
w/o bun	8 oz	570	40	63
Bean burrito	1	400	6	13
w/ sour cream		450	12	24
Bean curd & vegetable				
stir-fry	8 oz	180	13	65
Bean curd in peanut				
sauce w/ Chinese				
greens	10 oz	365	19	47
Black bean enchilada	1	445	20	41
Brown rice				
w/ peas, onions				
& Parmesan	8 oz	320	10	28
Brown vegetable rice	8 oz	370	24	58

	AMOUNT	CALORIES	FAT-GRAMS	% FAT
Calcutta Medley (soybeans, bulgur & brown rice w/ peanuts, apple, yogurt, curry)	8 oz	860	33	34
California casserole (brown rice, sour cream, cottage cheese, green chilies, cheddar)	8 oz	550	38	62
Chalupas (beans, tortilla, cheese, avocado, salsa	2 sm	325	18	50
Cheese & nut loaf (brown rice, cottage cheese, sesame seeds, peanuts, walnuts, wheat germ, eggs)	8 oz	525	42	72
Cheese enchilada	1	490	34	62
Chili relleno	1	340	24	64
Cottage cheese patties (cottage cheese, wheat germ, bread crumbs, walnuts, cream of mushroom soup)	2	440	30	62
Couscous w/ fruit	8 oz	450	16	32
Crusty Soybean Crowd-Pleaser (soybeans, corn, tomatoes, onion, wheat germ, Parmesan, brown rice)	8 oz	305	11	33

	AMOUNT	CALORIES	FAT-GRAMS	% FAT
Curried soybeans & peanuts over brown rice	8 oz	490	15	28
Curried stuffed pepper (millet, lentils, peas, mushrooms, carrots, almonds, cashews)	1	585	34	52
Dilled carrot cutlets (soybeans, carrots, peanuts, wheat germ, oil)	8 oz	355	23	58
East-West bean bake (brown rice, soybeans, wheat germ, mozzarella)	8 oz	265	13	49
Eggplant & cheese casserole	8 oz	215	14	58
Eggplant bake	8 oz	420	12	25
Eggs Grinnel (egg, spinach, cheese)	1 egg	215	15	62
Esau's Potage (brown rice, lentils, onions, celery, mushrooms)	8 oz	410	15	33
Falafel patties, broiled	8 oz	300	15	45
Golden parsley potatoes (potatoes, cottage cheese, cheddar)	8 oz	285	13	41
Leafy Chinese tofu (tofu, spinach, peanut oil)	8 oz	220	17	70
Legumes Continental (garbanzo beans, pinto beans, cabbage, cheddar)	8 oz	795	54	61

	AMOUNT	CALORIES	FAT-GRAMS	% FAT
Mexican bean stew	8 oz	220	4	16
Peanut sauce over vegetable salad	1 serving	445	31	62
Potato-bean bake (lentils, soybeans, mashed potatoes, mushrooms)	10 oz	440	22	45
Potatoes Gruyère	8 oz	365	19	47
Potato pancakes	2 cakes	495	13	24
Quesadilla (6")	1	245	16	58
Red & sweet curried rice	8 oz	445	13	26
Russian Surprise (navy beans, potatoes, onions, cucumber, sour cream, pumpernickel)	8 oz	520	20	35
Russian sweet cabbage	12 oz	325	10	28
Sesame vegetable rice (4 oz rice, 8 oz vegetables)	12 oz	545	29	48
Soybean soufflé	8 oz	135	9	60
Spinach-rice pot	8 oz	580	42	65
Spinach & tomato casserole	8 oz	135	7	46
Stuffed eggplant	1 slice	305	23	68
Summer squash & brown rice (w/ yogurt, Parmesan, egg, bread crumbs)	8 oz	230	14	54
Tostada w/ avocado	1	590	37	56
Vegetable paella	8 oz	635	23	32
Vegetable stew	8 oz	505	32	57

	AMOUNT	CALORIES	FAT-GRAMS	% FAT
Veggie burger				
w/ bun	6 oz	355	18	46
w/o bun	6 oz	225	16	64
Walnut-rice cheddar				
loaf	8 oz	590	42	64
Zucchini & cheddar				
casserole	8 oz	325	18	50
Zucchini bake	8 oz	105	5	43
Zucchini frittata	2 eggs	215	16	67
Zucchini-rice bake	8 oz	195	11	50

FAST-FOOD RESTAURANTS

The vast majority of foods offered at fast-food restaurants are rich in fat, so it makes good sense to visit these restaurants infrequently. If you do choose to eat fast food, be sure to eat low-fat foods at other meals to compensate.

General Tips

■ Make smart choices. The fast-food industry has responded to public pressure by offering more healthful items. For example, McDonald's has reduced the fat content of its shakes by about 80%, leaving only 1 or 2 grams of fat, and has introduced its McLean Deluxe Burger with 10 grams of fat. Burger King has also complied by cutting more than half the fat from its Broiler Chicken Sandwich. But the Double Western Bacon Cheeseburger at Carl's Jr. has 63 grams of fat and 1,030 calories, and the Taco Salad at Taco Bell has 61 grams of fat, and 905 calories each providing more fat in a single meal than most people should consume in an entire day.

SMART CHOICES	CALORIES	FAT-GRAMS	% FAT
Arby's Light Roast Chicken Deluxe	250	5	18
Wendy's Chili, regular size	220	7	29
Taco Bell Fiesta Tostada	170	7	38
Burger King B K Broiler Chicken Sandwich	270	8	27
McDonald's Small Hamburger	255	9	32
Wendy's Grilled Chicken Sandwich	320	9	25
Domino's 16" Cheese Pizza, 2 slices	375	10	24
Hardee's Roast Beef Sandwich	350	11	28

■ Watch out for added fat. Salad bars and prepackaged salads are healthy foods, but they can be turned into unhealthy choices with added fat. A prepackaged salad with chicken has only about 3 or 4 grams of fat, but top it with a 2-ounce package of ranch dressing and you'll add about 34 grams of fat. It's a far better idea to ask for diet or no-oil dressings. McDonald's Lite Vinaigrette, for instance, has just 2 grams of fat in each package.

■ When ordering breakfast, opt for pancakes and syrup (no butter or margarine) instead of breakfast sandwiches that combine cheese, egg and/or meat filling with a muffin, croissant or biscuit. This switch saves about 30 grams of fat.

■ Pizza can be a good bet if you order wisely. Pass up meat toppings such as pepperoni, ground beef and sausage, which drive up the fat content to the level of cheeseburgers. Order cheese pizza "with half the cheese, extra tomato sauce and more vegetables," and you'll have a fast food you can live with.

■ At Mexican fast-food outlets, order the plain bean burrito or tostada for less fat than the loaded versions—a plain bean burrito at Taco Bell will save you 10 grams of fat over a Burrito Supreme.

■ Think about preparation methods. The biggest problem is that most fast foods are fried, which means added fat-grams.

Burgers

■ Hamburgers are still America's favorite fast food. But not all hamburgers are the same, as shown in the table that follows.

BURGER	CALORIES	FAT-GRAMS	% FAT
Wendy's Single, plain	340	15	40
McDonald's Quarter Pounder	410	20	44
McDonald's Big Mac	500	26	47
Hardee's Big Deluxe Burger	500	30	54
Wendy's Big Classic	570	33	52
Burger King Whopper	615	36	53
Burger King Double Whopper w/ Cheese	935	61	59

■ Avoid croissant sandwiches. One croissant contains the equivalent of four pats of butter.

■ Many delis offer extra-lean corned beef, pastrami and beef brisket, but watch out for portion size. The sandwiches made with these meats are large enough to feed two people, so order a half-sandwich or split a whole one with a friend. Also, be careful with side dishes such as creamy coleslaw and/or potato salad.

■ High-fat sub sandwiches are those made with bologna, hard or Genoa salami, pepperoni, mortadella and cheese. Opt instead for turkey, smoked turkey, ham and lean roast beef. Avoid oil and mayonnaise in favor of mustard, onions, lettuce, pickles and hot peppers.

Fried Foods

■ Fried chicken is extremely high in fat—Kentucky Fried Chicken's "Extra Crispy" chicken is 21 grams. If you eat fried chicken, choose the breast and remove the skin and breading. Exercise portion control—limit yourself to one piece. Many of the complements are high in fat, such as coleslaw, onion rings and French fries. Choose corn on the cob, mashed potatoes or baked beans instead.

■ Chicken nuggets are battered and fried, so most of their calories come from fat. Six McDonald's McNuggets yield about 15 grams of fat.

■ Fried fish and seafood have the same basic problem as fried chicken. Avoid deep-fried fish, oysters, scallops, shrimp and clams. Unfortunately, fried seafood often comes with high-fat complements such as coleslaw or French fries. A good example is the Homestyle Fish Dinner at Long John Silver's (3 pieces of fish, fryes, coleslaw, and 2 hush puppies) with 39 grams of fat. Instead, choose low-fat items. Long John Silver's Baked Fish with Paprika (2 pieces) comes with rice pilaf and a side salad. The damage to your budget is only 2 grams of fat.

■ A typical medium serving of French fries has 17 grams of fat. Some chains offer baked potatoes with steamed vegetables as a low-fat alternative.

■ As size and number of patties increase, so does the fat. Single hamburgers have about 2 ounces of meat, quarter-pounders about 3 ounces, and triples 4 or more ounces. Order items identified as "small," "single" or "junior." Avoid those labeled "jumbo," "super," "double," "triple," "extra large" and "big."

■ Don't make the mistake of eating too many small burgers. There is no advantage in eating two Wendy's Junior hamburgers with a combined 18 grams of fat, for instance, over one Wendy's regular hamburger at 15 grams.

■ Watch out for fatty add-ons. Opt for a plain hamburger with lettuce, tomato, onion and ketchup (10 to 15 grams of fat) instead of the supreme version loaded with cheese, bacon, mayonnaise or mayo-based "special sauces" (50 to 60 grams of fat).

■ Roast beef sandwiches can be a good alternative to hamburgers. Stick with the regular or junior-size sandwich, and avoid high-fat extras such as mayonnaise, mayo-based sauces and cheese.

Sandwiches

■ Sandwiches can be a good choice or a disaster. Stick with low-fat sandwich fillers such as roasted turkey breast, roasted or grilled chicken breast, lean roast beef, and lean ham. Avoid cold cuts, tuna or chicken salads with mayonnaise, egg salad, cheese sandwiches and cheese melts.

■ The best choice for a chicken sandwich is a skinless, grilled breast. Watch out for sandwiches that use fried chicken—Burger King's Fried Chicken Sandwich has 40 grams of fat. As with other sandwiches, cut out the extras such as mayonnaise, mayo-based sauces, cheese, and cheese sauces.

■ A fried fish fillet sandwich is not a good choice. Breaded, fried in grease, and covered with mayonnaise and fatty sauces, it is an item to be avoided. Wendy's Fish Fillet Sandwich, for example, will set you back 29 fat-grams.

■ Watch out for fatty condiments on sandwiches. A Subway Roast Beef Sandwich without oil has about 10 grams of fat; with oil, it has over 17 grams. Use mustard, horseradish or ketchup to moisten the bread, but skip oil, butter, margarine or mayonnaise.

	AMOUNT	CALORIES	FAT-GRAMS	% FAT

ARBY'S*

Biscuits, Croissants & Muffins

	AMOUNT	CALORIES	FAT-GRAMS	% FAT
Biscuit, Plain	1	280	15	48
Bacon	1	320	18	51
Sausage	1	460	32	62
Croissant, Plain	1	260	16	54
Bacon & Egg	1	390	26	61
Ham & Cheese	1	345	21	54
Sausage & Egg	1	520	39	68
Muffin, Blueberry	1	200	6	25

Desserts

	AMOUNT	CALORIES	FAT-GRAMS	% FAT
Cheese Cake	1	305	23	57
Chocolate Chip Cookie	1	130	4	28
Cinnamon Nut Danish	1	340	9	25
Polar Swirls				
Butterfinger	1	460	18	36
Oreo	1	480	20	37
Peanut Butter	1	515	24	42
Snickers	1	510	19	33
Turnovers				
Apple	1	305	18	54
Blueberry	1	320	19	53
Cherry	1	280	18	57

Drinks & Shakes

	AMOUNT	CALORIES	FAT-GRAMS	% FAT
Coca-Cola, Medium	1	130	0	0
Small	1	95	0	0
Large	1	160	0	0
Hot Chocolate	1	110	1	10

Listings for Arby's and the chains in the following pages reflect standard servings.

	AMOUNT	CALORIES	FAT-GRAMS	% FAT
Milk, 2%	1	120	4	33
Orange Juice	1	80	0	0
Shakes				
Chocolate	1	450	12	23
Jamocha	1	370	10	26
Vanilla	1	330	11	31
Potatoes				
Baked, Plain	1	240	2	7
Broccoli & Cheddar	1	420	18	39
Butter/Margarine				
& Sour Cream	1	465	25	49
Deluxe	1	620	36	53
Mushroom				
& Cheese	1	515	27	47
Cakes	1 order	205	12	53
French Fries				
Small	1 order	245	13	48
Regular	1 order	395	21	48
Large	1 order	490	26	48
Cheddar	1 order	400	22	49
Curly	1 order	340	18	47
Salads & Salad Dressings				
Salads				
Cashew Chicken	1	590	37	56
Chef	1	220	10	44
Garden	1	110	5	43
Roast Chicken	1	170	7	35
Side	1	25	0	0
Dressings				
Blue Cheese	1	295	31	95
Buttermilk Ranch	1	350	38	99
Honey French	1	320	27	75
Light Italian	1	25	1	43
Thousand Island	1	300	29	88

ARBY'S

	AMOUNT	CALORIES	FAT-GRAMS	% FAT
Sandwiches				
Chicken				
Barbecue	1	380	14	34
Breast	1	490	26	47
Cordon Bleu	1	660	37	50
Fajita Pita	1	255	9	32
Grilled Deluxe	1	425	21	45
Light Roast Deluxe	1	255	5	17
Roast Club	1	515	29	51
Roast Deluxe	1	375	19	47
Fish Fillet	1	540	29	49
Ham & Cheese	1	330	14	38
Roast Beef				
Bac 'N Cheddar Deluxe	1	530	33	55
Beef 'N Cheddar	1	450	20	40
French Dip	1	345	12	32
French Dip 'N Swiss	1	425	18	39
Light Deluxe	1	295	10	30
Philly Beef 'N Swiss	1	500	26	47
Roast Beef, Regular	1	355	15	38
Junior	1	220	11	44
Giant	1	530	27	46
Super	1	530	28	48
Turkey Deluxe	1	400	20	46
Light Roast Deluxe	1	250	4	15
Sauces				
Arby's Sauce	1 oz	30	0	0
Horsey Sauce	1 oz	55	5	82
Soups				
Beef w/ Vegetables & Barley	1	95	3	26
Boston Clam Chowder	1	210	11	46
Cheese	1	290	19	59

	AMOUNT	CALORIES	FAT-GRAMS	% FAT
Chicken Noodle	1	100	2	16
Corn Chowder	1	195	11	49
Cream of Broccoli	1	180	8	40
French Onion	1	70	3	42
Split Pea w/ Ham	1	200	10	43
Tomato	1	85	1	16

BASKIN-ROBBINS

	AMOUNT	CALORIES	FAT-GRAMS	% FAT
Cone				
Sugar	1	60	1	15
Waffle	1	140	2	13
Frozen Yogurt				
Low-Fat				
Chocolate, Medium	1	245	7	26
Small	1	175	5	26
Large	1	315	9	26
Strawberry Vanilla,				
Medium	1	211	7	30
Small	1	150	5	30
Large	1	270	9	30
Nonfat				
Coconut, Medium	1	140	0	0
Small	1	100	0	0
Large	1	180	0	0
Raspberry, Medium	1	165	0	0
Raspberry, Strawberry				
Small	1	125	0	0
Large	1	225	0	0
Strawberry, Medium	1	175	0	0
Ice Cream				
Regular				
Chocolate	1 scoop	270	14	47
Chocolate Chip	1 scoop	260	15	52

	AMOUNT	CALORIES	FAT-GRAMS	% FAT
French Vanilla	1 scoop	280	18	58
Jamoca Almond Fudge	1 scoop	270	14	47
Pralines 'n Cream	1 scoop	280	14	45
Rocky Road	1 scoop	300	14	42
Strawberry	1 scoop	220	10	41
Vanilla	1 scoop	240	14	53
World Class Chocolate	1 scoop	280	14	45
Light				
Chocolate Caramel Nut	½ cup	130	5	35
Espresso & Cream	½ cup	120	5	38
Praline Dream	½ cup	130	6	42
Strawberry	½ cup	110	3	25
Sherbet & Sorbets				
Rainbow Sherbet	1 scoop	160	2	11
Red Raspberry Sorbet	1 scoop	140	0	0

BURGER KING

Bagels, Biscuits, Croissants & Muffins

	AMOUNT	CALORIES	FAT-GRAMS	% FAT
Bagels				
Bacon, Egg & Cheese Sandwich	1	455	20	40
Egg & Cheese Sandwich	1	410	16	35
Ham, Egg & Cheese Sandwich	1	440	17	35
Plain	1	270	6	20
w/ Cream Cheese	1	370	16	39
Sausage, Egg & Cheese Sandwich	1	625	36	52

	AMOUNT	CALORIES	FAT-GRAMS	% FAT
Biscuits				
Plain	1	330	17	46
w/ Bacon	1	380	20	48
w/ Bacon & Egg	1	465	27	52
w/ Sausage	1	480	29	55
w/ Sausage & Egg	1	570	36	57
Croissants				
Plain	1	180	10	50
Croissan'wich				
w/ Bacon, Egg & Cheese	1	360	24	60
w/ Egg & Cheese	1	315	20	57
w/ Ham, Egg & Cheese	1	345	21	55
w/ Sausage, Egg & Cheese	1	535	40	67
Mini Muffins				
Blueberry	1	290	14	43
Lemon Poppyseed	1	320	18	51
Raisin Oat Bran	1	290	12	37
Breakfast Dishes				
Scrambled Egg Platter	1	550	34	56
w/ Bacon	1	610	39	58
w/ Sausage	1	770	53	62
French Toast Sticks	1 order	500	29	52
Great Danish	1	500	40	72
Chicken & Fish				
BK Broiler Chicken Sandwich	1	270	8	27
Chicken Tenders	6 pcs	235	13	50
Fried Chicken Sandwich	1	685	40	53
Fish Filet	1	495	25	45

	AMOUNT	CALORIES	FAT-GRAMS	% FAT
Desserts				
Apple Pie	1	310	14	41
Danish Pastry				
Apple Cinnamon	1	390	13	30
Cheese	1	405	16	35
Cinnamon Raisin	1	450	18	36
Drinks				
Coke, Medium	1	265	0	0
Diet Coke, Medium	1	0	0	0
Milk				
2%	1	120	5	37
Whole	1	160	9	52
Orange Juice	1	80	0	0
Shakes, Regular				
Chocolate	1	325	10	28
Strawberry	1	395	10	23
Vanilla	1	335	10	27
Sprite, Medium	1	265	0	0
Hamburgers				
Bacon Double Cheeseburger	1	515	31	54
Bacon Double Cheeseburger Deluxe	1	590	39	59
Barbecue Bacon Double Cheeseburger	1	535	31	52
Cheeseburger	1	320	15	42
Cheeseburger Deluxe	1	390	23	53
Double Cheeseburger	1	485	27	50
Hamburger	1	270	11	36
Hamburger Deluxe	1	345	19	50
Mushroom Swiss Double Cheeseburger	1	475	27	51

	AMOUNT	CALORIES	FAT-GRAMS	% FAT
Whopper	1	615	36	53
w/ Cheese	1	705	44	56
Double, w/ Cheese	1	935	61	59

Potatoes & Onion Rings

French Fries

Regular	1	230	13	52
Medium	1	370	20	48
Onion Rings	1 order	340	19	50

Salads & Salad Dressings

Salads

Chef	1	180	9	46
Chunky Chicken	1	140	4	25
Garden	1	95	5	47
Side	1	25	0	0

Dressings (per packet)

Bleu Cheese	1	300	32	96
French	1	290	22	68
House	1	260	26	35
Light Italian	1	170	18	95
Olive Oil & Vinegar	1	310	33	96
Ranch	1	350	37	95
Thousand Island	1	290	26	81

Sauces (per packet)

BK Broiler Sauce	1	40	4	90

Dipping Sauces

Barbecue	1	35	0	0
Honey	1	90	0	0
Ranch	1	170	18	95
Sweet & Sour	1	45	0	0
Mayonnaise	2 tbsp	195	21	97
Mustard	1	5	0	0
Tartar Sauce	1	135	14	94

BURGER KING

	AMOUNT	CALORIES	FAT-GRAMS	% FAT

CARL'S JR.

Breakfast Foods

	AMOUNT	CALORIES	FAT-GRAMS	% FAT
Bacon	2 slices	45	4	80
Breakfast Burrito	1	430	26	54
Cinnamon Roll	1	460	18	35
Danish Pastry	1	520	16	28
English Muffin				
w/ Margarine	1	190	5	24
French Toast Dips				
(no syrup)	1 order	490	26	48
Hot Cakes				
w/ Margarine				
(no syrup)	1 order	510	24	42
Muffins				
Blueberry	1	340	9	24
Bran	1	310	7	20
Sausage Patty	1	190	18	85
Scrambled Eggs	1 order	120	9	68
Sunrise Sandwich	1	300	13	39
w/ Bacon	1	345	17	44
w/ Sausage	1	490	31	57

Chicken, Fish & Beef

	AMOUNT	CALORIES	FAT-GRAMS	% FAT
Charbroiler BBQ				
Chicken Sandwich	1	310	6	17
Charbroiler Chicken				
Club Sandwich	1	570	29	46
Country Fried Steak				
Sandwich	1	720	43	54
Fish Sandwich	1	560	30	48
Roast Beef Club				
Sandwich	1	620	34	49
Roast Beef Deluxe				
Sandwich	1	540	26	43

	AMOUNT	CALORIES	FAT-GRAMS	% FAT
Sante Fe Chicken Sandwich	1	540	13	22
Desserts				
Chocolate Chip Cookie	1	330	17	46
Fudge Brownie	1	430	19	40
Fudge Brownie Mousse Cake	1	400	23	52
Raspberry Cheesecake	1	310	17	49
Drinks & Shakes				
Carbonated Drink	1	240	0	0
Diet	1	0	0	0
Milk, 1%	1	140	2	30
Orange Juice, Small	1	90	1	10
Shake, Regular	1	350	7	18
Small	1	270	5	17
Large	1	460	9	18
Hot Dogs & Hamburgers				
All Star Hot Dog	1	540	35	58
Chili Dog	1	720	47	59
Hamburgers				
Carl's Original	1	460	20	39
Double Western Bacon Cheeseburger	1	1,030	63	55
Famous Star	1	610	38	56
Happy Star	1	320	14	39
Super Star	1	820	53	58
Western Bacon Cheeseburger	1	730	39	48
Potatoes & Onion Rings				
Baked Potatoes				
Bacon & Cheese	1	730	43	53
Broccoli & Cheese	1	590	31	47

	AMOUNT	CALORIES	FAT-GRAMS	% FAT
Cheese	1	690	36	47
Fiesta	1	720	38	48
Lite	1	290	1	3
Sour Cream & Chive	1	470	19	36
French Fries, Regular	1 order	420	20	43
Small	1 order	280	13	42
Large	1 order	545	26	43
Criss-Cut	1 order	330	22	60
Hash Brown Nuggets	1 order	270	17	57
Onion Rings	1 order	520	26	45

Salad & Salad Dressings

	AMOUNT	CALORIES	FAT-GRAMS	% FAT
Salad				
Charbroiler Chicken	1	200	8	36
Garden	1	50	3	54
Salad Dressings				
Blue Cheese	1	300	30	90
House	1	220	22	90
Italian	1	240	26	98
Reduced Calorie				
French	1	80	4	45
Thousand Island	1	220	22	90

Sauces (per packet)

	AMOUNT	CALORIES	FAT-GRAMS	% FAT
Guacamole	1	50	4	72
Salsa	1	10	0	0
Taco Sauce	1	10	0	0

CHURCH'S FRIED CHICKEN

Chicken

	AMOUNT	CALORIES	FAT-GRAMS	% FAT
Fried Breast	1	280	17	56
Fried Leg	1	150	9	53
Fried Thigh	1	305	22	65
Fried Wing	1	305	20	59
Nuggets	6 pcs	330	19	51

	AMOUNT	CALORIES	FAT-GRAMS	% FAT
Desserts				
Apple Pie	1	300	19	57
Pecan Pie	1	370	20	48
Fish				
Fried Catfish	3 pcs	200	12	54
Miscellaneous				
Coleslaw	1	85	7	76
Corn on the Cob, Buttered	1	165	3	18
Dinner Roll	1	85	2	17
French Fries, Regular	1	255	13	45
Hush Puppy	1	80	3	33

DAIRY QUEEN/BRAZIER

	AMOUNT	CALORIES	FAT-GRAMS	% FAT
Chicken & Fish				
Chicken Breast Fillet Sandwich	1	450	20	40
w/ Cheese	1	500	25	45
Chicken Nuggets	6 pcs	275	18	59
Fish Fillet Sandwich	1	390	16	37
w/ Cheese	1	440	21	43
Grilled Chicken Sandwich	1	300	8	24
Desserts				
Banana Split	1	540	11	18
Buster Bar	1	450	29	58
Dilly Bar	1	210	13	56
Frozen Yogurt, Vanilla	1	100	0	0
Fudge Nut Bar	1	405	25	55
Heath Blizzard	1	800	24	27
Hot Fudge Brownie Delight	1	600	25	38

	AMOUNT	CALORIES	FAT-GRAMS	% FAT
Parfait	1	430	8	17
Parfait, Peanut Butter	1	740	34	41
Soft Ice Cream Cones,				
Regular	1	240	7	26
Small	1	140	4	26
Large	1	340	10	26
Soft Ice Cream				
Cones, Dipped,				
Regular	1	340	16	42
Small	1	190	9	43
Large	1	510	24	42
Strawberry Shortcake	1	540	11	18
Sundae, Chocolate,				
Regular	1	310	8	23
Small	1	190	4	19
Large	1	440	10	20
Drinks & Shakes				
Float	1	410	7	15
Freeze	1	500	12	22
Malt, Chocolate,				
Regular	1	760	18	21
Small	1	440	10	21
Large	1	890	21	21
Mr. Misty				
Small	1	190	0	0
Regular	1	250	0	0
Large	1	340	0	0
Float	1	390	7	16
Freeze	1	500	12	22
Kiss	1	70	0	0
Shake, Chocolate,				
Regular	1	710	19	24
Small	1	410	11	24
Large	1	830	22	24

	AMOUNT	CALORIES	FAT-GRAMS	% FAT
Hamburgers & Hot Dogs				
Hamburger	1	330	13	35
w/ Cheese	1	380	18	43
Hamburger, Double	1	480	25	47
w/ Cheese	1	590	34	52
Hamburger, Triple	1	710	45	57
w/ Cheese	1	820	50	55
Hamburger, "Ultimate"	1	730	47	58
Hot Dog	1	280	16	51
w/ Cheese	1	340	21	56
w/ Chili	1	330	19	52
Hot Dog, Quarter Pound	1	480	36	68
w/ Cheese	1	535	40	68
w/ Chili	1	575	41	64
Potatoes & Onion Rings				
French Fries, Regular	1	210	10	43
Large	1	340	16	42
Onion Rings, Regular	1	240	12	45

DOMINO'S PIZZA

(Serving size: based on 16-inch pizza, thin crust, which serves 6.)

	AMOUNT	CALORIES	FAT-GRAMS	% FAT
Cheese Pizza	2 slices	375	10	24
Deluxe Pizza	2 slices	500	20	37
Double Cheese/ Pepperoni Pizza	2 slices	545	25	42
Ham Pizza	2 slices	420	11	24
Pepperoni Pizza	2 slices	460	17	34
Sausage/Mushroom Pizza	2 slices	430	16	33
Veggie Pizza	2 slices	500	10	36

	AMOUNT	CALORIES	FAT-GRAMS	% FAT

DUNKIN' DONUTS

Bagels

Cinnamon 'N Raisin	1	250	2	7
Egg	1	250	2	7
Onion	1	230	1	4
Plain	1	240	1	4

Croissants

Almond	1	420	27	58
Chocolate	1	440	29	59
Plain	1	310	19	55

Cookies

Chocolate Chunk	1	200	10	45
w/ Nuts	1	210	11	47
Oatmeal Pecan Raisin	1	200	9	41

Donuts & Cakes

Apple Filled Cinnamon Donut	1	190	9	43
Bavarian Filled Donut w/ Chocolate Frosting	1	240	11	41
Blueberry-Filled Donut	1	210	8	34
Boston Kreme Donut	1	240	11	41
Chocolate Frosted Yeast Ring	1	200	10	45
Glazed Buttermilk Ring	1	290	14	43
Glazed Chocolate Ring	1	325	21	58
Glazed Coffee Roll	1	280	12	39
Glazed French Cruller	1	140	8	51

	AMOUNT	CALORIES	FAT-GRAMS	% FAT
Glazed Whole Wheat Ring	1	330	18	49
Glazed Yeast Ring	1	200	9	41
Honey Dipped Cruller	1	260	11	38
Jelly Filled Donut	1	220	9	37
Lemon Filled Donut	1	260	12	42
Plain Cake Ring Donut	1	260	18	62
Powdered Cake Ring	1	270	16	53
Muffins				
Apple N' Spice	1	300	8	24
Banana Nut	1	310	10	29
Blueberry	1	280	8	26
Bran w/ Raisins	1	310	9	26
Corn	1	240	12	32
Oat Bran	1	330	11	30

GODFATHER'S PIZZA

Original				
Cheese, Medium	⅛ pie	270	8	27
Mini	¼ pie	190	4	19
Small	1/6 pie	240	7	26
Large (Hot Slice)	⅛ pie	370	11	27
Large	1/10 pie	300	9	27
Combo, Medium	⅛ pie	400	17	38
Mini	¼ pie	240	7	26
Small	1/6 pie	360	15	38
Large (Hot Slice)	⅛ pie	550	24	39
Large	1/10 pie	440	19	39
Thin Crust				
Cheese, Medium	⅛ pie	210	7	30
Small	1/6 pie	180	6	30
Large	1/10 pie	230	7	28

	AMOUNT	CALORIES	FAT-GRAMS	% FAT
Combo, Medium	⅛ pie	310	14	41
Small	⅙ pie	270	13	43
Large	¹/₁₀ pie	335	16	43

Stuffed Pie

	AMOUNT	CALORIES	FAT-GRAMS	% FAT
Cheese, Medium	⅛ pie	350	13	33
Small	⅙ pie	310	11	32
Large	¹/₁₀ pie	380	16	38
Combo, Medium	⅛ pie	480	23	43
Small	⅙ pie	430	20	42
Large	¹/₁₀ pie	520	26	45

HARDEE'S

Breakfast Foods

Big Country Breakfast

	AMOUNT	CALORIES	FAT-GRAMS	% FAT
w/ Bacon	1	660	40	55
w/ Ham	1	620	33	48
w/ Sausage	1	850	57	60
Fried Egg	1	80	6	74

Muffins

	AMOUNT	CALORIES	FAT-GRAMS	% FAT
Blueberry	1	400	19	43
Oat Bran Raisin	1	440	18	37
Pancakes	3	280	2	6
w/ 1 Sausage Patty	3	430	16	33
w/ 2 Bacon Strips	3	350	9	23

Biscuits

	AMOUNT	CALORIES	FAT-GRAMS	% FAT
Bacon	1	360	21	53
Bacon & Egg	1	410	24	53
Bacon, Egg & Cheese	1	460	28	55
Canadian Rise 'N' Shine	1	470	27	52
Chicken	1	430	22	46
Cinnamon 'N' Raisin	1	320	17	48
Country Ham	1	350	18	46
Country Ham & Eggs	1	400	22	50

	AMOUNT	CALORIES	FAT-GRAMS	% FAT
Ham	1	320	16	45
Ham & Egg	1	370	19	46
Ham, Egg & Cheese	1	420	23	49
'N' Gravy	1	440	24	49
Rise 'N' Shine	1	320	18	51
Sausage	1	440	28	57
Sausage & Egg	1	490	31	57
Steak	1	500	29	52
Steak & Egg	1	550	32	52
Chicken & Fish				
Chicken Fillet	1	370	13	32
Chicken Stix	6 pcs	210	9	39
Fisherman's Fillet	1	500	24	43
Fried Chicken				
Breast	1	410	24	52
Breast & Wing	1	605	37	55
Leg	1	140	8	51
Leg & Thigh	1	435	28	58
Thigh	1	295	20	61
Wing	1	190	13	61
Desserts				
Apple Turnover	1	270	12	40
Big Cookie	1	250	13	47
Cool Twist Cone				
Chocolate	1	200	6	27
Vanilla	1	190	6	28
Cool Twist Sundae				
Caramel	1	330	10	27
Hot Fudge	1	320	12	34
Strawberry	1	260	8	28
Frozen Yogurt				
Chocolate	1	170	4	21
Vanilla	1	160	4	23

HARDEE'S

	AMOUNT	CALORIES	FAT-GRAMS	% FAT
Drinks & Shakes				
Milk, 2%	1	120	4	33
Shakes				
Chocolate	1	460	8	16
Strawberry	1	440	8	16
Vanilla	1	400	9	20
Hamburgers & Hot Dogs				
Bacon Cheeseburger	1	610	39	58
Big Deluxe Burger	1	500	30	54
Cheeseburger	1	320	14	39
Deluxe Burger				
(The Lean 1)	1	420	18	39
Hamburger	1	270	10	33
Hot Dog	1	300	17	51
Mushroom 'N' Swiss				
Burger	1	490	27	50
Quarter-Pound				
Cheeseburger	1	500	29	52
Potatoes				
French Fries, Regular	1	230	11	43
Large	1	360	17	43
Crispy Curls	1	300	16	48
"Big Fry"	1	500	23	41
Hash Rounds	1 order	230	14	55
Salads & Salad Dressings				
Salads				
Chef	1	240	15	56
Chicken Fiesta	1	280	15	48
Garden	1	210	14	60
Side	1	20	0	0
Salad Dressings (per packet)				
Blue Cheese	1	210	18	77
House	1	290	29	90

	AMOUNT	CALORIES	FAT-GRAMS	% FAT
Reduced Calorie				
French	1	130	5	35
Reduced Calorie				
Italian	1	90	8	80
Thousand Island	1	250	23	83
Sandwiches				
Chicken Fillet Deli				
Supreme	1	380	14	33
Grilled Chicken	1	310	9	26
Grilled Chicken				
Supreme	1	320	10	28
Ham 'N' Cheese Deli				
Supreme	1	390	17	39
Hot Ham 'N' Cheese	1	330	12	33
Roast Beef	1	350	11	28
w/ Cheese	1	405	15	33
Roast Beef, Large	1	375	12	29
w/ Cheese	1	430	17	36
Roast Beef Deli				
Supreme	1	370	17	41
Turkey Club	1	390	16	37
Turkey Club				
Supreme	1	390	16	37
Sauces (per packet)				
Barbecue Sauce	1	15	0	0
Dipping Sauce				
BBQ	1	30	0	0
Honey	1	45	0	0
Sweet Mustard	1	50	0	0
Sweet 'n' Sour	1	40	0	0
Horseradish	1	25	2	75
Mayonnaise	1	50	5	90
Tartar Sauce	1	90	9	90

HARDEE'S

	AMOUNT	CALORIES	FAT-GRAMS	% FAT

JACK IN THE BOX

Breakfast

	AMOUNT	CALORIES	FAT-GRAMS	% FAT
Breakfast Jack	1	310	13	38
Canadian Crescent	1	450	31	62
Pancake Platter	1	610	22	32
Sausage Crescent	1	585	43	66
Scrambled Egg Platter	1	560	32	52
Scrambled Egg Pocket	1	430	21	44
Supreme Crescent	1	545	40	66

Chicken, Turkey & Fish

Chicken Fajita Pita	1	290	8	25
Chicken Strips	6 pcs	450	20	40
Chicken Supreme	1	640	39	55
Fish Supreme	1	510	27	48
Grilled Chicken Fillet	1	410	17	38
Ham & Turkey Melt	1	590	36	55

Desserts

Cheesecake	1	310	18	51
Double Fudge Cake	1	290	9	28
Hot Apple Turnover	1	350	19	49

Drinks & Shakes

Coca-Cola Classic,				
Regular	1	145	0	0
Large	1	385	0	0
Diet Coke	1	0	0	0
Dr Pepper, Sprite	1	145	0	0
Iced Tea	1	0	0	0
Milk Shakes				
Chocolate	1	330	7	19
Strawberry	1	320	7	20
Vanilla	1	320	6	17
Milk, 2%	1	120	5	37

	AMOUNT	CALORIES	FAT-GRAMS	% FAT
Orange Juice	1	80	0	0
Ramblin' Root Beer	1	175	0	0
Hamburgers				
Bacon Cheeseburger	1	705	45	57
Cheeseburger	1	315	14	40
Double Cheeseburger	1	470	27	52
Grilled Sourdough Burger	1	710	50	63
Ham & Swiss Burger	1	640	39	54
Hamburger	1	270	11	37
Jumbo Jack	1	585	34	52
w/ Cheese	1	680	40	53
Old Fashioned Patty Melt	1	715	46	58
Miscellaneous				
Cheese Nachos	1 order	570	35	55
Club Pita	1	285	8	27
Egg Rolls	5 pcs	755	41	49
Guacamole	1 pkg	55	5	82
Sirloin Cheesesteak	1	620	30	43
Super Taco	1	280	17	54
Taco	1	190	11	53
Potatoes & Onion Rings				
French Fries, Regular	1 order	350	17	44
Small	1 order	220	11	45
Jumbo	1 order	395	19	43
Seasoned Curly	1 order	360	20	50
Hash Browns	1 order	155	11	63
Onion Rings	1 order	380	23	54
Salads & Salad Dressings				
Salads				
Chef	1	325	18	50
Pasta Seafood	1	395	22	50

	AMOUNT	CALORIES	FAT-GRAMS	% FAT
Side	1	50	3	53
Taco	1	505	31	55
Salad Dressings				
(per packet)				
Bleu Cheese	1	260	22	76
Buttermilk House	1	360	36	90
Reduced Calorie				
French	1	175	8	41
Thousand Island	1	310	30	87

KENTUCKY FRIED CHICKEN

Chicken

Breast				
Chargrill	1	240	13	49
Extra Tasty Crispy	1	340	20	52
Lite 'n Crispy	1	220	12	49
Original Recipe	1	285	15	49
Drumstick				
Chargrill	1	105	6	50
Extra Tasty Crispy	1	205	14	61
Lite 'n Crispy	1	120	7	52
Original Recipe	1	145	8	52
Hot Wings	6 pcs	375	24	58
Kentucky Nuggets	6 pcs	275	17	57
Side Breast				
Extra Tasty Crispy	1	345	22	59
Lite 'n Crispy	1	205	12	55
Original Recipe	1	270	16	56
Thigh				
Chargrill	1	170	12	63
Extra Tasty Crispy	1	405	30	66
Lite 'n Crispy	1	245	17	61
Original Recipe	1	295	20	60

	AMOUNT	CALORIES	FAT-GRAMS	% FAT
Wing				
Chargrill	1	120	8	60
Extra Tasty Crispy	1	255	19	66
Original Recipe	1	180	12	59
Desserts				
Parfait				
Apple Shortcake	1	275	10	33
Chocolate Creme	1	360	19	48
Fudge Brownie	1	330	11	30
Lemon Creme	1	515	20	36
Strawberry Shortcake	1	230	9	34
Pudding				
Chocolate	1	155	7	43
Vanilla	1	160	7	41
Miscellaneous				
Baked Beans	1 order	135	2	11
Buttermilk Biscuit	1	235	12	45
Cole Slaw	1 order	120	7	50
Corn on the Cob	1	175	3	16
French Fries	1 order	245	12	44
Mashed Potatoes and Gravy	1 order	70	2	20
Nugget Sauce (per packet)				
Barbecue	1	35	1	15
Honey	1	50	0	0
Mustard	1	35	1	23
Sweet 'n Sour	1	60	1	9
Potato Salad	1 order	180	12	59
Sandwiches				
Chicken Lites	1	170	10	54
Colonel's Chicken	1	480	27	51
Colonel's Chicken Deluxe	1	550	32	53

	AMOUNT	CALORIES	FAT-GRAMS	% FAT

LONG JOHN SILVER'S

Chicken

	AMOUNT	CALORIES	FAT-GRAMS	% FAT
Baked Chicken	1	140	4	26
Baked Chicken Sandwich (no sauce)	1	320	8	23
Chicken Nuggets Dinner	6 pcs	700	45	58
Chicken Plank	1 pc	130	6	42
Chicken Planks Dinner	4 pcs	1,040	59	51
Chicken Sandwich, Batter-Dipped (no sauce)	1	440	17	35

Desserts

	AMOUNT	CALORIES	FAT-GRAMS	% FAT
Apple Pie	1	320	13	37
Cherry Pie	1	360	13	33
Lemon Pie	1	340	9	24
Pecan Pie	1	530	25	42

Fish & Shellfish

	AMOUNT	CALORIES	FAT-GRAMS	% FAT
Catfish Fillet	1 pc	180	11	55
Clams				
Breaded	1 order	240	12	45
Dinner	1	955	58	55
Cod				
Baked	1 pc	130	0	0
Delight	1 pc	180	1	5
Supreme	1 pc	190	4	19
Fish				
Battered	1 pc	210	12	51
Dinner, Fried, 3 pieces	1	1,180	70	53
Homestyle	1 pc	125	7	50

	AMOUNT	CALORIES	FAT-GRAMS	% FAT
Fish & Fryes				
2 pieces	1	650	36	50
3 pieces	1	850	48	51
Fish Sandwich				
Batter-Dipped				
(no sauce)	1	380	16	38
Homestyle	1	510	22	39
Oysters, Breaded	1 pc	60	3	45
Scallop Dinner	1	750	45	54
Seafood Platter	1	975	58	53
Shrimp				
Battered	1 pc	60	4	60
Batter-Fried Dinner	1	710	45	57
Breaded	1 order	190	10	47
Breaded Shrimp				
Platter	1	960	57	53
Homestyle	1 pc	45	3	60
Scampi, Baked	1 order	160	7	39
Miscellaneous				
Baked Potato				
(no topping)	1	150	0	0
Breadstick, Fried	1	110	3	25
Clam Chowder	1 order	130	5	35
Cole Slaw, drained				
on fork	1 order	140	6	39
Corn Cobette	½ ear	140	8	51
French Fryes	1 order	170	6	32
Green Beans	1 order	30	0	0
Hushpuppies	1 pc	70	2	26
Rice Pilaf	1 order	210	2	9
Seafood Chowder				
w/ Cod	1 order	140	6	39
Seafood Gumbo				
w/ Cod	1 order	120	8	60

	AMOUNT	CALORIES	FAT-GRAMS	% FAT
Tartar Sauce	1 pkt	70	3	39
Vegetables	1 order	120	6	45
Salads & Salad Dressings				
Salads				
Garden	1	170	9	48
Ocean Chef	1	150	5	30
Seafood	1	230	5	20
Side	1	25	0	0
Salad Dressings (per packet)				
Bleu Cheese	1	120	2	15
Lite Italian	1	12	0	0
Ranch	1	90	2	20
Sea Salad	1	90	4	40

McDONALD'S

Breakfast

	AMOUNT	CALORIES	FAT-GRAMS	% FAT
Biscuits				
w/ Bacon, Egg & Cheese	1	430	26	54
w/ Biscuit Spread	1	260	13	45
w/ Sausage	1	420	28	60
w/ Sausage & Egg	1	500	33	59
Breakfast Burrito	1	280	17	55
Cheerios	¾ cup	80	1	11
Danish				
Apple	1	390	17	39
Cinnamon Raisin	1	440	21	43
Iced Cheese	1	390	21	48
Raspberry	1	410	16	35
English Muffin w/ Margarine	1	170	5	26
Hotcakes w/ Margarine & Syrup	1 order	410	9	20

	Amount	Calories	Fat-Grams	% Fat
McMuffin				
Egg	1	280	11	35
Sausage	1	345	20	52
Sausage w/ Egg	1	415	25	54
Muffins				
Apple Bran, Fat Free	1	180	0	0
Blueberry, Fat Free	1	170	0	0
Pork Sausage	1 order	180	16	82
Sausage	1 order	160	15	84
Scrambled Eggs	1 order	140	10	64
Wheaties	¾ cup	90	1	10
Chicken & Fish				
Chicken Fajitas	1 order	185	8	39
Chicken McNuggets	6 pcs	270	15	50
Filet-O-Fish	1	370	18	44
Grilled Chicken Breast				
Sandwich	1	250	4	14
McChicken	1	415	20	43
Desserts				
Apple Pie	1	260	15	52
Cherry Pie	1	260	14	47
Chocolaty Chip Cookies	1	330	16	43
Frozen Yogurt				
Cone, Vanilla, Low-Fat	1	105	1	7
Sundae, Hot Caramel, Low-Fat	1	270	3	9
Sundae, Hot Fudge, Low-Fat	1	240	3	12
Sundae, Strawberry, Low-Fat	1	210	1	5
Hot Caramel Sundae	1	340	9	24
Hot Fudge Sundae	1	310	9	26

McDONALD'S

	AMOUNT	CALORIES	FAT-GRAMS	% FAT
McDonaldland Cookies	1 order	290	9	29
Orange Sorbet Ice				
Cone	1	105	2	0
Sundae (no topping)	1	140	0	0
Orange Sorbet Ice/				
Low-Fat Frozen				
Yogurt				
Twist Cone	1	105	1	4
Twist Sundae	1	140	1	3
Drinks & Shakes				
Apple Juice	1	90	0	0
Coca-Cola Classic,				
Regular	1	140	0	0
Large	1	380	0	0
Diet Coke	1	0	0	0
Grapefruit Juice	1	80	0	0
Milk, 1%	1	110	1	16
Milk Shake				
Chocolate Low-Fat	1	320	2	5
Strawberry Low-Fat	1	320	1	4
Vanilla Low-Fat	1	290	1	4
Orange Drink	1	130	0	0
Orange Juice	1	80	0	0
Sprite	1	140	0	0
Hamburgers				
Big Mac	1	500	26	47
Cheeseburger	1	305	13	38
Hamburger	1	255	9	32
McD.L.T.	1	580	37	57
McLean Deluxe	1	320	10	28
w/ Cheese	1	370	14	34
Quarter Pounder	1	410	20	49
w/ Cheese	1	510	28	72

	AMOUNT	CALORIES	FAT GRAMS	% FAT
Miscellaneous				
Carrot Sticks	1 order	40	0	0
Celery Sticks	1 order	15	0	0
Hot Mustard				
Sauce	1 pkt	70	4	46
McRib Sandwich	1	445	22	44
Potatoes				
French Fries, Medium	1 order	320	17	48
Small	1 order	220	12	49
Large	1 order	400	22	50
Hash Browns	1 order	130	7	48
Salads & Salad Dressings				
Salads				
Chef	1	170	9	48
Chunky Chicken	1	150	4	24
Garden	1	50	2	36
Side	1	30	1	30
Salad Dressings				
(per packet)				
Bleu Cheese	1	250	20	72
Lite Vinaigrette	1	48	2	38
Peppercorn	1	400	44	98
Ranch	1	220	20	82
Red French Reduced-				
Calorie	1	160	8	45
Thousand Island	1	390	40	92

PIZZA HUT

Hand-Tossed Pizza, Medium

Cheese	2 slices	520	20	35
Pepperoni	2 slices	500	23	41
Supreme	2 slices	540	26	43
Super Supreme	2 slices	555	25	40

	AMOUNT	CALORIES	FAT-GRAMS	% FAT
Pan Pizza, Medium				
Cheese	2 slices	490	18	33
Pepperoni	2 slices	540	22	37
Supreme	2 slices	590	30	46
Super Supreme	2 slices	565	26	42
Personal Pan Pizza, Whole				
Pepperoni	1	675	29	39
Supreme	1	650	28	39
Thin 'n Crispy Pizza, Medium				
Cheese	2 slices	400	17	38
Pepperoni	2 slices	415	20	44
Supreme	2 slices	460	22	43
Super Supreme	2 slices	465	21	41

ROY ROGERS

	AMOUNT	CALORIES	FAT-GRAMS	% FAT
Breakfast				
Biscuit	1	230	12	47
Crescent Roll	1	290	18	56
Crescent Sandwich	1	400	27	61
w/ Bacon	1	430	30	63
w/ Ham	1	445	29	59
w/ Sausage	1	450	29	58
Egg & Biscuit Platter	1	395	27	62
w/ Bacon	1	435	30	62
w/ Ham	1	440	29	59
w/ Sausage	1	460	29	57
Pancake Platter				
w/ Bacon	1	495	18	33
w/ Ham	1	505	17	30
w/ Sausage	1	610	30	44
w/ Syrup & Butter	1	450	15	30

	AMOUNT	CALORIES	FAT-GRAMS	% FAT
Chicken				
Breast	1	410	24	52
Breast & Wing Combo	1	605	37	55
Drumstick	1	140	8	51
Nuggets	6	270	17	57
Thigh	1	295	20	61
Thigh & Leg Combo	1	435	28	58
Wing	1	190	13	61
Desserts				
Brownie	1	265	11	38
Danish				
Apple	1	250	12	43
Cheese	1	255	12	43
Cherry	1	270	14	47
Strawberry Short				
Cake	1	450	19	38
Sundaes				
Caramel	1	295	9	28
Hot Fudge	1	340	13	35
Strawberry	1	215	7	29
Drinks & Shakes				
Coke, Regular	1	145	0	0
Diet Coke, Regular	1	0	0	0
Hot Chocolate	1	125	2	15
Milkshake				
Chocolate	1	360	10	25
Strawberry	1	315	10	29
Vanilla	1	305	11	32
Hamburgers				
Bacon Cheeseburger	1	580	39	60
Cheeseburger	1	565	37	59
Hamburger	1	455	28	55
RR Bar Burger	1	610	39	57

ROY ROGERS

	AMOUNT	CALORIES	FAT-GRAMS	% FAT
Potatoes				
French Fries, Regular	1 order	270	14	47
Large	1 order	360	18	45
Hot Topped Potato	1	210	0	0
w/ Bacon & Cheese	1	400	22	50
w/ Broccoli & Cheese	1	375	18	43
w/ Margarine	1	275	7	23
w/ Sour Cream & Chives	1	410	21	46
w/ Taco Beef & Cheese	1	465	22	43
Salads & Salad Dressings				
Salads				
Cole Slaw	2 tbsp	50	3	54
Macaroni Salad	2 tbsp	60	4	60
Potato Salad	2 tbsp	50	3	54
Salad Dressings				
Bacon & Tomato	2 tbsp	135	12	79
Bleu Cheese	2 tbsp	150	16	96
Low-Cal Italian	2 tbsp	70	6	77
Ranch	2 tbsp	155	14	81
Thousand Island	2 tbsp	160	16	90

SHAKEY'S PIZZA

	AMOUNT	CALORIES	FAT-GRAMS	% FAT
Homestyle				
Cheese	1 slice	305	14	42
Mushroom & Sausage	1 slice	345	17	45
Onion, Green Peppers, Olives & Mushrooms	1 slice	320	15	42
Pepperoni	1 slice	345	15	39
Pepperoni & Sausage	1 slice	375	20	48
Shakey's Special	1 slice	385	21	49

	AMOUNT	CALORIES	FAT-GRAMS	% FAT
Thick Crust				
Cheese	1 slice	170	5	27
Green Peppers, Black Olives & Mushrooms	1 slice	160	4	22
Pepperoni	1 slice	185	6	29
Pepperoni & Sausage	1 slice	180	8	41
Sausage & Mushroom	1 slice	180	6	30
Shakey's Special	1 slice	210	8	35
Thin Crust				
Cheese	1 slice	135	5	34
Onion, Green Peppers, Black Olives & Mushrooms	1 slice	125	5	36
Pepperoni	1 slice	150	7	43
Pepperoni & Sausage	1 slice	165	8	43
Sausage & Mushroom	1 slice	140	6	38
Shakey's Special	1 slice	170	9	47

SUBWAY

	AMOUNT	CALORIES	FAT-GRAMS	% FAT
Salads				
Chef, Small	1	190	10	47
Garden	1	45	0	10
Ham, Small	1	170	10	53
Roast Beef, Small	1	185	10	49
Seafood & Crab, Small	1	200	11	51
Tuna, Small	1	210	12	49
Turkey, Small	1	170	9	50
Sandwiches (6-inch)				
Ham	1	360	11	28
Meatball	1	430	16	34
Roast Beef	1	375	11	26
Seafood & Crab	1	390	12	29

	AMOUNT	CALORIES	FAT-GRAMS	% FAT
Steak	1	425	14	30
Subway Club	1	380	11	26
Tuna	1	400	13	28
Turkey	1	360	10	26

TACO BELL

Burritos

Bean w/ Red Sauce	1	450	14	28
Beef w/ Red Sauce	1	500	21	38
Chicken (no sauce)	1	335	12	32
Combination	1	410	16	35
Fiesta	1	225	9	36
Supreme w/ Red Sauce	1	505	22	39

Miscellaneous

Chilito	1	385	18	42
Cinnamon Twists	1	170	8	42
Enchirito w/ Red Sauce	1	380	20	47
Mexican Pizza	1	575	37	58
Meximelt				
Beef	1	265	15	51
Cheese	1	260	15	53
Nachos	1 order	350	18	47
Bellgrande	1 order	650	35	49
Supreme	1 order	370	27	66

Salads, Salad Dressings & Sauces

Salads				
Chicken Salad	1	125	8	58
Taco w/ Shell	1	905	61	61
Taco w/o Shell	1	485	31	58
Salad Dressing, Ranch	1 pkt	235	25	95
Sauces				
Green Sauce	1	5	0	0
Guacamole	1	35	2	53

	AMOUNT	CALORIES	FAT-GRAMS	% FAT
Hot Taco Sauce	1 pkt	5	0	0
Pico de Gallo	1	10	0	0
Red Sauce	1	10	0	0
Salsa	1	20	0	0
Sour Cream	1	45	4	78
Taco Sauce	1 pkt	5	0	0
Taco				
Beef				
Hard Shell	1	185	11	54
Soft Shell	1	225	12	48
Bellgrande	1	335	23	62
Chicken				
Hard Shell	1	170	9	47
Soft Shell	1	215	10	42
Downsized Taco	1	130	7	50
Soft Taco	1	150	7	43
Steak, Soft Shell	1	220	11	45
Supreme	1	230	15	59
Supreme, Soft Shell	1	270	16	53
Tostada				
Beef w/ Red Sauce	1	245	11	41
Chicken w/ Red Sauce	1	265	15	51
Fiesta	1	170	7	38

TCBY (THE COUNTRY'S BEST YOGURT)

Nonfat Frozen Yogurt				
Kiddie	1	90	0	0
Small	1	160	0	0
Regular	1	225	0	0
Large	1	290	0	0
Super	1	420	0	0
Giant	1	870	0	0

	AMOUNT	CALORIES	FAT-GRAMS	% FAT
Regular Frozen Yogurt				
Kiddie	1	95	2	23
Small	1	180	4	23
Regular	1	245	6	23
Large	1	315	8	23
Super	1	460	11	23
Giant	1	950	24	23
Sugar-Free Frozen Yogurt				
Kiddie	1	65	0	0
Small	1	120	0	0
Regular	1	165	0	0
Large	1	210	0	0
Super	1	305	0	0
Giant	1	630	0	0

WENDY'S

	AMOUNT	CALORIES	FAT-GRAMS	% FAT
Breakfast				
Bacon	2 slices	110	10	82
Breakfast Sandwich	1	370	19	46
Danish	1	360	18	45
French Toast	2 slices	400	19	43
Omelet				
Ham & Cheese	1	250	17	61
w/ Mushroom	1	290	21	65
Mushroom, Onion &				
Green Pepper	1	210	15	64
Sausage	1 patty	200	18	81
Sausage & Gravy	1 order	440	36	74
Scrambled Eggs	1 order	190	12	57
Chicken & Fish				
Chicken Club Sandwich	1	505	25	44
Chicken Sandwich, Fried	1	430	19	40

	AMOUNT	CALORIES	FAT-GRAMS	% FAT
Crispy Chicken				
Nuggets	6 pcs	280	20	64
Fish Filet Sandwich	1	460	25	49
Grilled Chicken				
Sandwich	1	320	9	25
Desserts				
Chocolate Chip				
Cookie	1	275	23	43
Frosty Dairy Dessert,				
Medium	1	520	18	32
Small	1	400	14	32
Large	1	680	24	32
Pudding				
Butterscotch	1	90	4	40
Chocolate	1	90	4	40
Drinks				
Chocolate Milk	1	160	5	28
Coca-Cola,				
Medium	1	150	0	0
Small	1	100	0	0
Large	1	200	0	0
Biggie	1	350	0	0
Diet Coke, Small	1	0	0	0
Dr Pepper, Small	1	100	0	0
Hot Chocolate	1	110	1	8
Lemonade	1	90	0	0
Lemon-Lime	1	100	0	0
Milk, 2%	1	110	4	33
Hamburgers				
Big Classic	1	570	33	52
w/ Cheese	1	640	39	55
Double	1	750	45	54
Double w/ Cheese	1	820	51	56

	AMOUNT	CALORIES	FAT GRAMS	% FAT
Cheeseburger	1	410	21	46
Double	1	590	33	50
w/ Bacon	1	460	28	55
Hamburger, Plain	1	340	15	40
Double, Plain	1	520	27	47
w/ Everything	1	420	21	45
Jr. Burgers				
Bacon Cheeseburger	1	430	25	52
Cheeseburger	1	310	13	38
Hamburger	1	260	9	31
Swiss Deluxe	1	360	18	45
Miscellaneous				
Chicken Fried Steak	1	580	41	64
Chili, Regular	1 order	220	7	29
Large	1 order	360	12	30
New Chili	1 order	230	9	35
Potatoes				
Baked, Plain	1	270	0	0
Hot Stuffed Bacon & Cheese	1	520	18	31
Hot Stuffed Broccoli & Cheese	1	400	16	36
Hot Stuffed Cheese	1	420	15	32
Hot Stuffed Chili & Cheese	1	500	18	32
Hot Stuffed Sour Cream & Chives	1	500	23	42
French Fries				
Small	1 order	240	12	32
Large	1 order	310	16	45
Biggie	1 order	450	22	45
Home Fries	1 order	360	22	55

	AMOUNT	CALORIES	FAT-GRAMS	% FAT

Salads, Salad Dressings & Salad Bar
(Average servings unless otherwise indicated)

	AMOUNT	CALORIES	FAT-GRAMS	% FAT
Alfalfa Sprouts	1	10	0	0
Alfredo Sauce	1	35	1	26
Applesauce, Chunky	1	20	0	0
Bacon Bits	1	40	2	45
Bananas	1	25	0	0
Breadsticks	2	30	1	30
Broccoli, Fresh, ½ cup	1	10	0	0
Cantaloupe, Fresh	1	20	0	0
Carrots, Fresh, ¼ cup	1	10	0	0
Cauliflower, Fresh, ½ cup	1	15	0	0
Cheddar Chips, 1 oz	1	160	12	68
Cheese				
Cheddar, Shredded	1	110	10	82
Cheese Sauce	1	40	2	46
Cottage	1	110	4	33
Imitation, Shredded	1	90	6	60
Parmesan, Grated, 1 oz	1	130	9	62
Chicken Salad	1	120	8	60
Cole Slaw, 2 oz	1	70	5	64
Croutons, ½ oz	1	60	3	45
Cucumbers, Fresh, 4 slices	1	5	0	0
Fettuccine	1	190	3	14
Flour Tortilla	1	110	3	25
Garbanzo Beans	1	45	1	20
Garlic Toast	1	70	3	39
Green Peppers, Fresh, ¼ cup	1	10	0	0
Lettuce, 1 cup	1	10	0	0
Mushrooms, Fresh, ¼ cup	1	5	0	0

WENDY'S

	AMOUNT	CALORIES	FAT-GRAMS	% FAT
Olives, Black	1	35	3	77
Oranges, Fresh, 2 oz	1	25	0	0
Pasta Medley, 2 oz	1	60	2	30
Pasta Salad, ¼ cup	1	35	0	0
Peaches, in Syrup, 2 pcs	1	30	0	0
Pepperoni, Sliced, 1 oz	1	140	12	77
Potato Salad, ¼ cup	1	125	11	79
Refried Beans	1	70	3	39
Rotini	1	90	2	20
Salad Dressings				
(4 tbsps)				
Blue Cheese	1	360	40	100
Celery Seed	1	280	18	58
French	1	240	24	90
Golden Italian	1	180	16	80
Hidden Valley Ranch	1	200	24	100
Italian Caesar	1	320	36	100
Reduced Calorie				
Bacon & Tomato	1	180	16	80
Reduced Calorie				
Italian	1	100	8	72
Sweet Red French	1	280	24	77
Thousand Island	1	280	28	90
Salads				
Chef	1	180	9	45
Garden	1	100	5	44
Taco	1	660	37	50
Seafood	1	110	7	57
Sauces				
Alfredo	2 tbsp	50	2	36
Cheese	2 tbsp	50	2	36
Picante	2 oz	20	0	0
Spaghetti	2 tbsp	40	0	0
Sour Cream	1	60	6	90

	AMOUNT	CALORIES	FAT-GRAMS	% FAT
Sour Topping	1	60	5	78
Imitation, 1 oz	1	45	4	80
Spaghetti Sauce	1	30	0	0
w/ Meat, 2 oz	1	60	2	30
Spanish Rice	1	70	1	13
Sunflower Seeds &				
Raisins, 1 oz	1	140	10	64
Taco Chips, 2 oz	1	260	10	35
Taco Meat	1	110	7	57
Taco Shell	1	45	3	60
Tartar Sauce, 1 tbsp	1	120	14	100
Three Bean Salad,				
¼ cup	1	60	0	0
Tuna Salad	1	100	6	54

WHATABURGER

Breakfast

Breakfast on a Bun	1	520	34	59
Egg Omelette Sandwich	1	310	15	43
Pancakes	1 order	200	3	13
w/ Sausage	1 order	410	22	48
Pecan Danish	1	270	16	52
Sausage	1 order	150	9	54

Drinks & Shakes

Orange Juice	1	85	0	0
Vanilla Shake, Small	1	320	9	25

Hamburgers

Whataburger	1	580	24	37
w/ Cheese	1	670	33	44
Whataburger Junior	1	305	14	40
w/ Cheese	1	350	18	46
Justaburger	1	265	12	39
w/ Cheese	1	310	16	45

	AMOUNT	CALORIES	FAT-GRAMS	% FAT
Potatoes & Onion Rings				
French Fries, Regular	1 order	330	18	49
Small	1 order	220	12	49
Hash Browns	1 order	150	9	54
Onion Rings	1 order	225	12	49

WHITE CASTLE

	AMOUNT	CALORIES	FAT-GRAMS	% FAT
Breakfast				
Sausage & Egg Sandwich	1	320	12	62
Sausage Sandwich	1	195	8	55
Chicken & Fish				
Chicken Sandwich	1	185	8	39
Fish Sandwich	1	155	5	29
w/ 1 tbsp Tartar Sauce	1	230	12	47
Hamburgers				
Cheeseburger	1	200	11	50
Hamburger	1	160	8	45
Potatoes & Onion Rings				
French Fries, Regular	1 order	300	15	45
Onion Rings, Regular	1 order	245	13	48

	AMOUNT	CALORIES	FAT-GRAMS	% FAT

GENERIC FAST FOODS

	AMOUNT	CALORIES	FAT-GRAMS	% FAT
Breakfast				
Biscuit	1	275	13	42
Croissant				
w/ egg & cheese	1	370	25	60
w/ egg, cheese & bacon	1	415	28	62
w/ egg, cheese & ham	1	475	34	64
w/ egg, cheese & sausage	1	525	38	65
Danish				
Cheese	1	355	25	63
Cinnamon	1	350	17	43
Fruit	1	335	16	43
English muffin				
w/ butter	1	190	6	27
w/ cheese & sausage	1	395	24	56
w/ egg, cheese & Canadian bacon	1	385	20	47
w/ egg, cheese & sausage	1	490	31	57
French toast				
w/ butter	2 slices	360	19	47
Sticks	5	480	29	55
Hash brown potatoes	½ cup	150	9	54
Omelet, ham & cheese, 2 eggs	1 order	255	18	62
Pancakes w/ syrup & butter	3	520	14	24
Sausage	1 patty	100	8	72
Scrambled eggs	2	200	15	68

	AMOUNT	CALORIES	FAT-GRAMS	% FAT
Chicken				
Breaded & fried				
Dark meat	2 pcs	430	27	56
Wing & breast	2 pcs	495	30	54
Fillet w/o mayo	1	515	29	51
w/ cheese	1	630	39	55
Nuggets, plain	1 pc	50	3	54
	6 pcs	290	18	55
w/ barbecue				
sauce	6 pcs	330	18	49
w/ honey	6 pcs	330	18	48
w/ mustard sauce	6 pcs	325	19	53
w/ sweet & sour				
sauce	6 pcs	345	19	47
Desserts				
Brownie	1	245	10	37
Fried pie	1	265	14	47
Ice-cream cone,				
medium	1	230	7	27
Small	1	110	3	25
Large	1	340	10	27
Ice-cream cone dipped				
in chocolate,				
medium	1	300	13	39
Small	1	150	7	42
Large	1	450	20	40
Ice-cream sandwich	1	140	4	26
Soft-service ice cream				
w/ cone	1 oz	165	6	33
Sundae				
Carmel	1	305	9	27
Hot fudge	1	285	9	27
Strawberry	1	270	8	26

	AMOUNT	CALORIES	FAT-GRAMS	% FAT
Fish				
Clams, breaded & fried	¾ cup	450	26	52
Crab, soft shell, fried	1	335	18	48
Crabcake				
Baked	1	90	1	10
Fried	1	290	19	58
Fish fillet, battered/ breaded, fried	1	210	11	47
w/ tartar sauce & cheese	1	525	29	49
Oysters, battered/ breaded, fried	6	370	18	44
Scallops, breaded, fried	6	385	19	44
Shrimp, breaded, fried	6–8	455	25	49
Hamburgers & Hot Dogs				
Cheeseburger w/o mayo or mayo-type dressing, regular	1	320	15	42
Double	1	545	28	46
Large	1	610	33	49
Hamburger w/o mayo or mayo-type dressing, regular	1	275	12	39
Double	1	460	22	43
Large	1	511	27	48
Hot dog, regular	1	240	15	54
w/ chili	1	325	18	49
Corn dog	1	460	19	37
Mayo or mayo-type dressing	1 tbsp	100	11	100

	AMOUNT	CALORIES	FAT-GRAMS	% FAT
Mexican Food				
Burritos				
Bean	2	450	14	27
Bean & cheese	2	380	12	28
Bean & chili peppers	2	415	15	32
Bean & meat	2	510	18	32
Bean, cheese & beef	2	330	13	35
Beef	2	525	21	36
Beef & chili peppers	2	425	16	35
Beef, cheese & red chili peppers	2	635	25	35
Chili con carne	1 cup	255	8	28
Chimichanga				
Beef	1	425	20	42
Beef & cheese	1	445	24	48
Beef & red chili peppers	1	420	19	40
Beef, cheese & red chili peppers	1	360	18	43
Enchilada				
Cheese & beef	1	325	18	49
Cheese & sour cream	1	320	19	53
Cheese, beef & bean	1	345	16	42
Frijoles w/ cheese	1 cup	225	8	31
Nachos				
Cheese	6–8	345	19	49
Cheese & jalapeño pepper	6–8	610	34	50
Cheese, ground beef, beans & jalapeño pepper	6–8	570	30	49
Taco				
Small	1	370	21	51
Large	1	570	32	51

	AMOUNT	CALORIES	FAT-GRAMS	% FAT
Taco salad				
w/ chili con carne	1.5 cups	290	13	41
w/ ground beef & cheese	1.5 cups	280	15	47
Tostada				
Bean & cheese	1	225	10	40
Bean, beef & cheese	1	335	17	46
Beef & cheese	1	315	16	46
Beef, cheese & guacamole	2	360	23	58

Pizza

	AMOUNT	CALORIES	FAT-GRAMS	% FAT
Cheese, 12"	1 pie	875	20	21
	⅛ pie	110	3	24
Meat & vegetable, 12"	1 pie	1,215	35	26
	⅛ pie	150	4	24
Pepperoni, 12"	1 pie	1,080	42	35
	⅛ pie	135	5	33
Supreme, 10"				
Thick & chewy	½ pie	640	22	31
Thin & crispy	½ pie	510	21	37

Potatoes & Onion Rings

	AMOUNT	CALORIES	FAT-GRAMS	% FAT
Onion rings	8–9	175	16	80
Baked potato				
w/ cheese	1	475	29	54
w/ cheese & bacon	1	450	26	52
w/ cheese sauce & broccoli	1	400	21	47
w/ cheese sauce & chili	1	480	22	41
w/ sour cream & chives	1	395	22	50
French fries, regular	1 order	240	12	46
Large	1 order	360	19	47

	Amount	Calories	Fat-Grams	% Fat
Mashed, w/ whole				
milk & margarine	⅓ cup	65	1	14
Potato chips	1 oz	150	10	60

Salads & Dressings

Salads

	Amount	Calories	Fat-Grams	% Fat
Chef	1.5 cups	270	16	54
Coleslaw	½ cup	90	8	80
Tossed, no dressing	1.5 cups	30	0	0
w/ cheese	1.5 cups	100	6	51
w/ chicken	1.5 cups	105	2	17
w/ pasta & seafood	1.5 cups	380	21	49
w/ shrimp	1.5 cups	110	2	16
Macaroni	½ cup	170	6	32
Potato	½ cup	160	9	51
Waldorf	½ cup	90	5	50

Salad dressings

	Amount	Calories	Fat-Grams	% Fat
Blue cheese	1 pkg	340	34	90
French	1 pkg	230	21	81
Italian	1 pkg	325	34	94
Low-calorie	1 pkg	50	2	36
Oriental	1 pkg	100	1	9
Thousand Island	1 pkg	395	39	89
Wine vinegar	1 pkg	5	0	0

Sandwiches

	Amount	Calories	Fat-Grams	% Fat
Bacon, lettuce & tomato	1	290	16	50
Bologna w/o mayo	1	305	16	47
Chicken club	1	570	26	41
Chicken salad	1	255	20	71
Chicken, sliced	1	310	15	44
Corned beef	1	295	10	30
Cream cheese & jelly	1	370	16	39
Egg salad	1	285	13	41

	AMOUNT	CALORIES	FAT-GRAMS	% FAT
Ham w/o mayo	1	285	16	51
Ham & cheese w/o mayo	1	390	24	55
Ham salad	1	320	17	48
Liverwurst w/o mayo	1	260	12	42
Peanut butter	1	350	20	51
Peanut butter & jelly	1	385	15	35
Roast beef w/o mayo	1	345	14	36
w/ cheese	1	400	18	40
Sirloin steak (3 oz)	1	325	12	33
Submarine, 6–8″				
w/ roast beef & mayo	1	410	13	28
w/ salami, ham & cheese	1	455	19	37
Tuna salad	1	585	28	43
Tuna	1	400	19	43
Turkey w/o mayo	1	275	14	46

QUICK REFERENCE GUIDE

FAVORITE FOOD	AMOUNT	CALORIES	FAT-GRAMS	% FAT

QUICK REFERENCE GUIDE

FAVORITE FOOD	AMOUNT	CALORIES	FAT-GRAMS	% FAT

QUICK REFERENCE GUIDE

FAVORITE FOOD	AMOUNT	CALORIES	FAT-GRAMS	% FAT

QUICK REFERENCE GUIDE

FAVORITE FOOD	AMOUNT	CALORIES	FAT-GRAMS	% FAT

QUICK REFERENCE GUIDE

FAVORITE FOOD	AMOUNT	CALORIES	FAT-GRAMS	% FAT

QUICK REFERENCE GUIDE

FAVORITE FOOD	AMOUNT	CALORIES	FAT-GRAMS	% FAT

ABOUT THE AUTHORS

Joseph C. Piscatella is the author of three widely acclaimed books, *Don't Eat Your Heart Out, Choices for a Healthy Heart* and *Controlling Your Fat Tooth,* which have been enthusiastically endorsed by health professionals. His recovery from open-heart surgery at age 32 and successful approach to healthy lifestyle changes are welcome news to those interested in improving health.

President of the Institute for Fitness and Health, Inc., in Tacoma, Washington, Mr. Piscatella lectures on lifestyle management skills to a variety of clients, including Fortune 500 companies, professional associations, educational institutions and health professionals. His seminar has been cited in *Time* magazine for its effectiveness.

As a spokesperson for a healthy lifestyle, Mr. Piscatella is a frequent guest on television and radio, contributes to national publications, and has hosted a television series on making healthy lifestyle changes. He is a member of the American Association for Cardiopulmonary Rehabilitation, the Association for Fitness in Business and the National Wellness Association.

Bernie Piscatella is vice president of the Institute for Fitness and Health and is responsible for all the recipes and nutritional analysis in their books.

For information on Mr. Piscatella's lifestyle seminars, please contact:

Institute for Fitness and Health, Inc.
P.O. Box 98882
Tacoma, WA 98499
Tel. (206) 584-4481
FAX 206 584 6204